NIZIĆ / WALL & BALL THEORY

I M P R E S S U M

KUNA (Croatian word for *marten*) is a small, inquisitive and clever animal. What is more, the pine marten is a Croatian national symbol. Three semicircles on the tail represent three full decades of Croatian sovereignty (1991–2025). Under the *KUNA Label* MEDICINARIUM publishes innovative books from any scientific field, especially biomedicine. The books under this label bring new insights and perspectives into science.

Dinko Nizić, MD, PhD
Wall & Ball Theory:
A Small CT Study of
TT-TIM Distance

PUBLISHER • COVER & LAYOUT
MEDICINARIUM d.o.o.
Josipa Jurja Strossmayera 28/2
35000 Slavonski Brod
Republic of Croatia (Croatia)

EMAIL:
medicinarium.publishing@gmail.com

REVIEWERS
Mario Josipović, MD, PhD
orthopedic surgeon
Marko Šimunović, MD, PhD
clinical radiologist

PROOFREADING
Dinko Nizić, MD, PhD

PRINT
LIBRI PLUREOS GmbH
Friedensallee 273
22763 Hamburg
Federal Republic of Germany

Parts of the cover and Figures 7, 10, 11, 14, 29, 49, and 51 are based on graphic material freely available at *www.freepik.com* (Freepik Company, S. L., 13 Molina Lario Street, 5th floor, 29015 Málaga, Spain).

Place of Publication: Slavonski Brod
Year of Publication: 2025
Sign-off Date: 2025-10-21

CIP data is available in the computer catalog of the National and University Library in Zagreb under the number 001284161.

ISBN
978-953-46656-4-0 (paperback edition)

Dinko Nizić, MD, PhD

Wall & Ball Theory

A Small CT Study of TT-TIM Distance

300 pages
62 figures
50 tables
75 references

MEDICINARIUM

Contents

Foreword

The knee is the largest and one of the most complex joints in the human body. It is, therefore, not surprising that much of musculoskeletal research and clinical practice focuses on this joint, with insights and methodologies often extrapolated to other joints. Within the knee, the patellofemoral joint occupies a special place. Despite its relatively young age in phylogenetic terms and its intricate anatomy and biomechanics, it has long remained underrepresented in research compared with other compartments of the knee.

Functionally, the patellofemoral joint acts both as a system of load distribution and as a mechanical lever. By increasing the distance of the quadriceps tendon from the joint axis, the patella amplifies extensor force. The articular cartilage is uniquely adapted to withstand high compressive stresses. Yet, this elegant mechanism is highly sensitive to misalignment, muscular imbalance, and structural variation, rendering it particularly vulnerable to pathological overload and instability.

A clear understanding of these conditions is essential for effective management, whether by conservative measures such as physiotherapy and pharmacologic treatment, or by surgical approaches aimed at restoring alignment and stability. Because of the complexity of patellofemoral biomechanics and the multitude of contributing variables, there is a constant need to *simplify* diagnostic approaches and to develop more precise, independent tools for patient categorization and treatment planning.

This book takes an important step along that very path. Rather than attempting to survey the entirety of patellofemoral pathology, the author focuses on a single radiologic parameter: the tibial tuberosity–tibial intercondylar midpoint (TT-TIM) distance. By narrowing the scope, he achieves a depth of analysis that is rarely found in broader overviews. Through a meticulous examination of TT-TIM distance and its relationship to patellar instability, the book offers clinicians a potentially superior and independent measurement that could quite likely replace less robust and often interdependent indices currently in use.

The book is written as the unique synthesis of patellofemoral biomechanics, radiology and statistics. The statistical sections are written with clarity and accessibility, engaging even those who are not statistically inclined, while still stimulating for readers who enjoy methodological debate. Importantly, the author underscores that statistical significance alone is **never** sufficient to justify clinical action; only the magnitude and practical relevance of an effect can guide meaningful improvement in patient outcomes. This emphasis on *practical* significance is the hallmark of the work, bridging the gap between theoretical insight and clinical application.

'Wall & Ball Theory' also highlights the crucial importance of *measurement precision*. The author demonstrates that even with a well-defined indicator, accurate and reproducible measurements are essential for drawing meaningful conclusions. He carefully delineates the techniques used to standardize TT-TIM distance measurement, underscoring the importance of minimizing variability and ensuring the reliability of the data.

In my view, this book can serve readers both as a guide to the anatomy and biomechanics of the patellofemoral joint and as an introduction to a rigorous, clinically relevant statistical approach. Most importantly, it provides a *new*, *precise*, and *independent diagnostic tool*—one with immediate application in the clinical setting.

Mario Josipović, MD, PhD

Department of Orthopedic Surgery
University Hospital Center Zagreb
School of Medicine
Šalata 6–7

Signs & Abbreviations

%	percentage
&	ampersand ('and')
–	minus (negative; subtraction)
–/+	direction of rotation; negatives and positives
+	plus (positive; summing)
$<$	less than
=	equal
$>$	greater than
≈	approximately equal
≤	equal or less than
≥	equal or greater than
×	multiplied
†	excluded (zero) ranks
∑	(Greek capital letter 'sigma') sum
°	degrees
|d|	absolute difference
3D	three-dimensional
95% CI	95% confidence interval
A, B	study units
AUC	area under the curve
B_1	patellar apex

B_2	middle of the inferior part of the quadriceps tendon on the tibial tuberosity
C	Celsius
c	cut-off
CAT	computed axial tomography
Ch	chapter
cm	centimeter
CT	computed tomography
CV	coefficient of variation (the measure of imprecision)
d	difference
d_i	rank difference
d_i^2	squared rank difference
EA	extension angle
e.g.	(Latin 'exempli gratia') for example
et al.	(Latin 'et alter') and others
F	female; femur; force; frontal plane
Fig.	figure
FPR	false positive rate
FR	femoral rotation (angle)
FR-TR	→ KR
FTD	femoral trochlear dysplasia
FTR	→ TITO
ICC	intraclass correlation coefficient
i.e.	(Latin 'id est') that is
Int Orthop.	International Orthopaedics (orthopedic scientific journal)

IS	Insall-Salvati (ratio)
JLCA	joint line convergence angle
K	Kelvin
kg	kilogram
KR	knee rotation (angle)
L	lateral; left (knee; side); leg
LPTS	lateral plateau posterior tibial slope (angle)
l_R	length of the inferior part of the quadriceps tendon during relaxation of the quadriceps mechanism
l_{MVIC}	length of the inferior part of the quadriceps tendon during MVIC of the quadriceps mechanism
M	magnitude; male
m	Poisson's coefficient (3 : 4)
MAL	mechanical axis of the knee/leg
max	maximum
min	minimum
mm	millimeter
MPTS	medial plateau posterior tibial slope (angle)
MR	magnetic resonance
MRI	magnetic resonance imaging
MVIC	maximum voluntary isometric contraction (of the quadriceps mechanism)
n	number of measurements; sample size (participants; knees)

n^2	squared sample size
o	origin (of the orthogonal coordinate system)
P	probability (value)
Pr	probability
p.	page
PCL	posterior cruciate ligament
pp.	pages
PY	patellar yaw (according to Nove-Josserand and Dejour)
Q	quadriceps belly; quadriceps muscle; quadriceps mechanism
q	quadriceps vector
qt	quadriceps belly tangent (lateral; medial)
r	correlation coefficient; relationship of interest; rotation
R	relaxation (of the quadriceps mechanism); right (knee)
RA	'Roman arch'
ROC	receiver operating characteristic (curve)
ROI	region of interest
S	sagittal plane; South Pole; total rank sum
SA	sulcus angle
sd	standard deviation (the measure of imprecision)

Se	sensitivity
Sp	specificity
t	translation
T	calculated T (the smaller sum of W^- and W^+ ranks); transverse (axial) plane
TA-GT	tubérosité tibiale antérieure–gorge de la trochlée → TT-TG
Tc	critical T
TG	(femoral) trochlear groove (point)
TIM	tibial intercondylar midpoint
TITO	tibial torsion (angle) (at the level of the tibial tuberosity)
TLA	tibial longitudinal axis
TPR	true positive rate
TR	tibial rotation (angle)
TT	tibial tuberosity
TT-ME	tibial tuberosity–midepicondyle (distance)
TT-MIELTI	tibial tuberosity–mid inter-epicondyle trochlea intersection (distance)
TT-PCL	tibial tuberosity–posterior cruciate ligament (distance)
TT-RA	tibial tuberosity–Roman arch (distance)
TT-TG	tibial tuberosity–trochlear groove (distance)

TT-TIM	tibial tuberosity–tibial intercondylar midpoint (distance) (*indicator*)
TTT	tibial tuberosity transfer
TY	tendon yaw (according to Šimunović)
Var	variance (the measure of imprecision)
W	sum of signed ranks of difference
XR	X-rays (radiography)
x-y-z	axes (of the orthogonal coordinate system)
y_r	rotation around the *y*-axis
z_r	rotation around the *z*-axis (yaw)
α	(Greek small letter 'alpha') the level of statistical significance
Δl	difference between l_{MVIC} and l_R
ε	(Greek small letter 'epsilon') tendon strain
μ	(Greek small letter 'mu') arithmetic mean
ρ	(Greek small letter 'rho') Spearman's rank correlation coefficient (also: r_s); correlation magnitude
ρc	critical ρ
σ	(Greek small letter 'sigma') → sd
Φ	(Greek capital letter 'phi') transverse diameter of the leg
φ	(Greek small letter 'phi') transverse diameter of the quadriceps belly

In politics,
the key word is
control.

In statistics,
the key word is
uncertainty.

In clinical research,
the key word is
magnitude.

To my late father,
a mechanical engineer.

Introduction

In this small CT study, the orthopedic charts and CT images of 15 participants (n = 15) were retrospectively reviewed, each having two knees, one negative (–) and one positive (+), after confounders were excluded. Therefore, the cohort was a handful of carefully sifted natural – / + knee pairs. In addition, to accommodate for small sample size, I have used:

- higher statistical significance level, $\alpha = .01$ (to increase statistical power)*
- *Wilcoxon signed-rank test* (to test for differences) and *Spearman's* ρ (Greek small letter 'rho'; elsewhere r_s) (to test for correlations) (Šošić, 2004, pp. 340–2, 424),** calculated as:

$$\rho = 1 - \frac{6 \times \sum_{i=1}^{n} d_i^2}{n^3 - n} = 1 - \frac{6 \times \sum_{i=1}^{n} d_i^2}{n \times (n^2 - 1)}, \text{ where}$$

$$d_i = \rho(x_i) - \rho(y_i),\ -1 \leq \rho \geq 1.$$

The critical T and ρ values at 2-tailed $\alpha < .01$ are shown in the table (Stangroom, 2025; Altman, 1999, pp. 530 –1: Appendix B, Tables B8 and B9). If, for a given n, *calculated T* (the *lower* rank sum) was *lower than or equal* to the *critical T* (Tc), and if *calculated rho* (ρ) was *higher* than the *critical rho* (ρc), the result was statistically significant at < .01.

* This is in line with recent suggestions to change the level of statistical significance from .05 to .005, that is to say, .01 (Benjamin *et al.*, 2018).

** These two statistical tests were named after Frank Wilcoxon (1892–1965), an Irish American chemist and statistician, and Charles Edward Spearman (1863–1945), an English psychologist and statistician.

n	Tc	ρc
	.01	*.01*
6	—	.9429
7	—	.8929
8	0	.8571
9	1	.8167
10	3	.7818
11	5	.7455
12	7	.7273
13	9	.6978
14	12	.6747
15	15	.6536
16	19	.6324
17	23	.6152
18	27	.5975
19	32	.5825
20	37	.5684
21	42	.5545
22	48	.5426
23	54	.5306
24	61	.5200
25	68	.5100
26	75	.5002
27	83	.4915
28	91	.4828
29	100	.4744
30	109	.4665

n............ sample size (total number of pairs for Wilcoxon signed-rank test)

ρc......... critical value of ρ

Tc......... critical value of T

The main finding of any scientific study, however, should be the *magnitude* (*the size*) *of an effect for the relationship of interest.* In daily clinical practice, only practically important magnitudes are considered for clinical management. In statistical terms, this would mean a magnitude ≥ .80 for differences (d) and ≥ .50 for correlations (r) (Cohen, 1988, pp. 26, 81) (Fig. 1).* For Wilcoxon signed-rank test, the size of an effect (d) for the relationship of interest was a ratio of sum of signed ranks of difference, W, and the total rank sum, S, calculated simply as d = W / S (Cline, 2019, p. 74; Kerby, 2014, p. 5; Glantz, 2005, p. 379).** For Spearman's ρ, the size of an effect for the relationship of interest was the value of the calculated ρ.

The pivotal achievement of a scientific study is to find a *practical* effect for the relationship of interest. Statistical significance, though widely appreciated, does not offer the information a researcher *really* wants to know, and that is how *important* is the relationship of interest one has set to investigate.

* Theoretical importance belongs to academia whereas practical importance belongs to daily clinical practice. In the words of Cohen: 'If he (the investigator) anticipates it (the *difference*) to be *large*, he might posit *d* as .8 or 1.0.' and 'Thus, when an investigator anticipates a degree of *correlation* between two different variables "about as high as they come", this would by our definition be a *large* effect, r = .50.' Jacob Cohen (1923–1998) was a renowned American psychologist and statistician.

** There are different ways to calculate the effect size when Wilcoxon signed-rank test is used. The most widely known is $r = z/\sqrt{n}$ due to Rosenthal, 1991, p. 28. However, it would require *n* of at least 25 to ascertain the symmetric distribution of the rank sums. Moreover, it depends on the sample size as well as sample inequality, and may produce values outside the –1, +1 range.

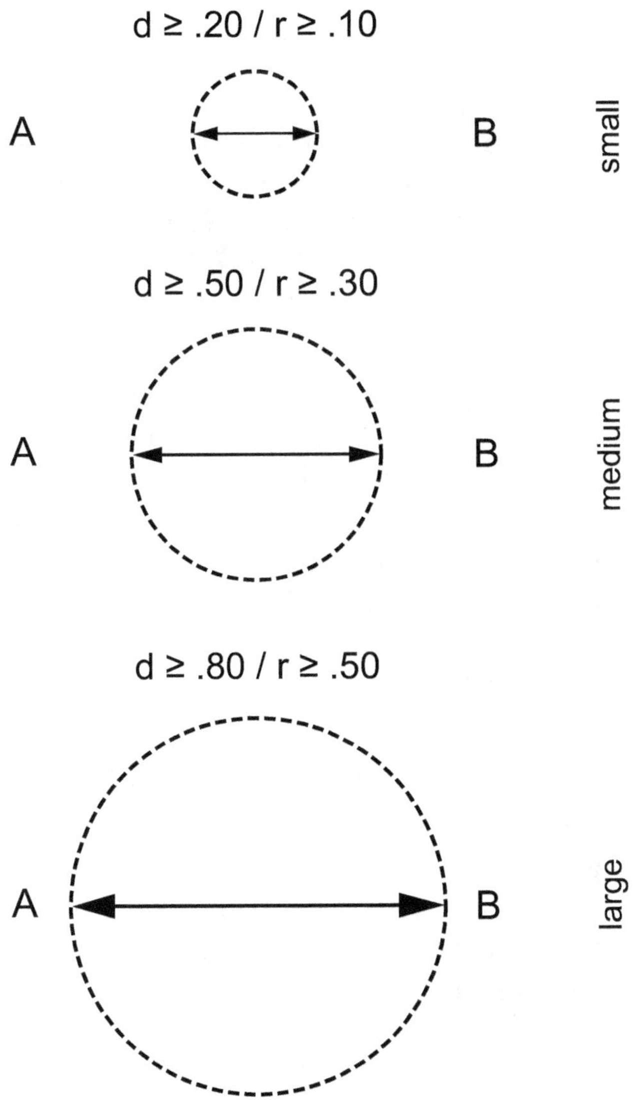

Fig. 1. The magnitudes

It is, therefore, crucial to understand the magnitude of an effect for the relationship of interest is *more* important than the statistical significance for the relationship of interest. How so?

Let us say one has found a small effect (≥.10) that is not statistically significant at < .01 in a sample n_1. The effect is not statistically significant because the sample is too small and cannot register such a small effect. In order to detect it, however, one could calculate the sample size required to confirm that particular magnitude, and increase the sample size by collecting a larger sample, n_2 ($n_2 > n_1$). The question here, however, is not a statistical, yet a logical one: *why* would anyone do it? * In the context of daily clinical practice, only large magnitudes are *practically* important. Small magnitudes are *theoretically* important. Why, then, would anyone spend additional resources such as time and money to prove statistical significance of an effect one knows beforehand is purely theoretical? The magnitudes for the relationship of interest are thought not to depend on the sample size either (Morris and Fritz, 2013, p. 580). So, to keep things in perspective, the first result one needs to look at is the magnitude of an effect for the relationship of interest. If that magnitude is small, and the relationship is not statistically significant, one should not bother collecting a larger sample as it represents a practically pointless vaste of resources (Fig. 2).

* Truth be told, it depends on the research field. For example, a study of a poisonous effect of a drug could be interested in very small changes in dosage, that is to say, a small effect size. In patellar stability research, this, however, is not as needed provided a sample is representative and, hence, reflects the true variability of the relationship of interest in the population.

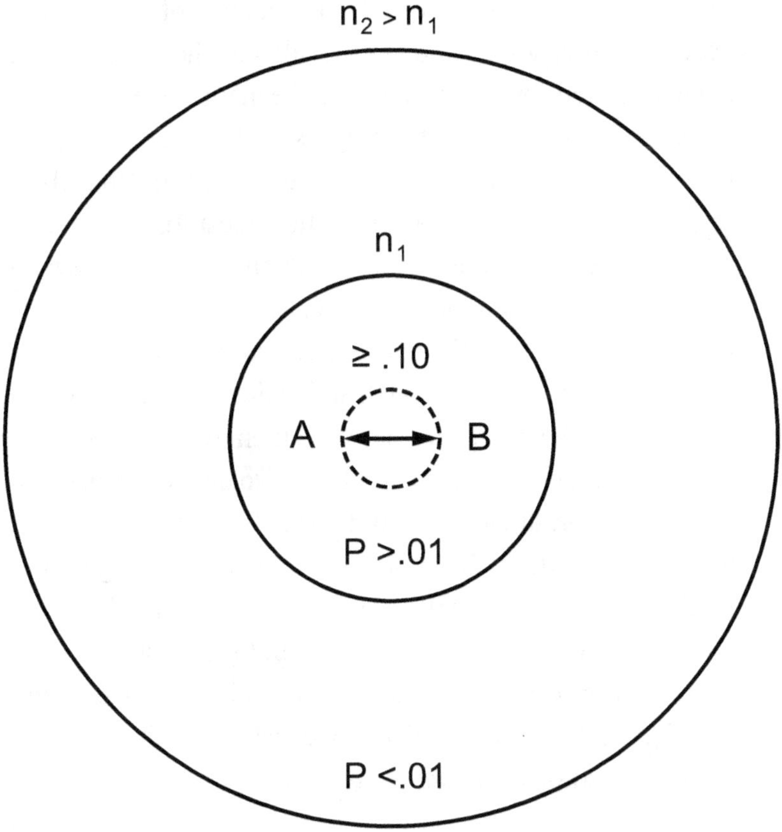

A, B ....study units
n_1 .... size of sample 1
n_2 .... size of sample 2
P .... probability (value)

Fig. 2. The relationship between the magnitude and the sample size if the magnitude were small

Apart from other scientific venues such as *astronomy*, magnitudes (M) are mainly reported in the context of *earthquakes*.* More recently, however, one has realized what empirical data have indicated some time ago, that the magnitude *does indeed change* with the change of a sample size. In fact, the magnitude is often *exaggerated* when the sample is small, and the relationship of interest is statistically significant resulting, on average, with *inflated* magnitudes which is a phenomenon called *type M error* or *exaggeration ratio* (Bertoldo *et al.*, 2022, p. 3; Gelman and Carlin, 2014, p. 643; Ioannidis, 2008, p. 640). If one would imagine a sample of only black and white balls, the magnitude of the effect, the *difference* between them will be *large*. If one decides to collect a larger sample yet also including black balls that are ¼ white and white balls that are ¼ black, the magnitude will *decrease*. If, furthermore, one collects even larger sample further including the balls that are half black and half white, the magnitude will *decrease* again, but would still be detectable mostly due to only black and only white balls in the sample (Fig. 3). So: the more *variability* one includes in the sample, the more magnitudes will *decrease*.

* The most famous earthquake scale is the *Richter magnitude base-10 logarithmic scale*, ranging from 1 to 10, devised by an American physicist Charles Francis Richter (1900–1985) in 1935, using an increase of wave amplitudes to gauge the effect. The earthquakes with the magnitude less than half, that is to say *less than 5* are considered *small*. This is similar to the interpretation of statistical magnitudes for relationships of interest where less than r = .50 would be regarded as *theoretical*.

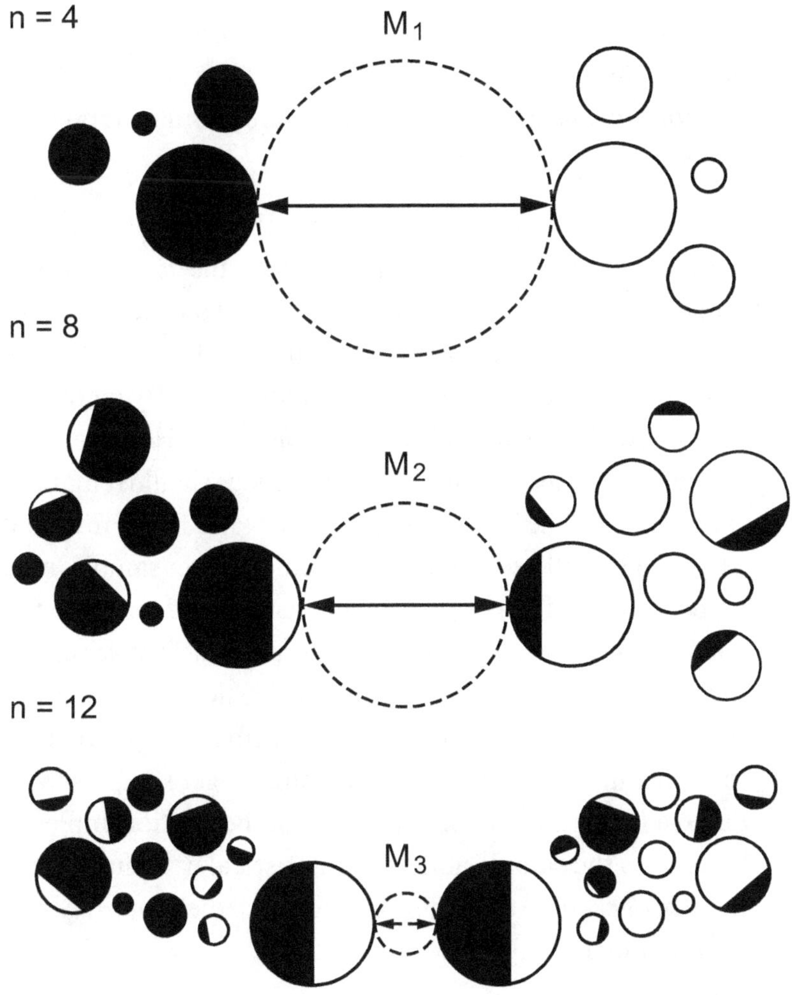

M_1, M_2, M_3......magnitudes
n.....................sample size

Fig. 3. Decrease in magnitudes with increasing sample size

One needs to understand a threshold estimate is an *arbitrary* variable, starting with Cohen's d $\geq$ .80 and r $\geq$ .50, the conventional use of which, it appears, Cohen himself did not advocate (Schäfer and Schwarz, 2019, p. 3). They are more or less *intuitional*, and should serve as a crude estimate if no other benchmarks were available.

Also, one needs to understand that in the midst of numerous magnitudes in this small CT study, it is not the *absolute* value* of the magnitude that is of interest here, but its *relative* stance with regard to other magnitudes. In other words: **the *ranking* of magnitudes is the key finding of the study**. By increasing the sample size, all magnitudes will *decrease*. However, their interpretation, the *hierarchy* of magnitudes should remain the same (Fig. 4). The largest magnitude one has found in a small sample will still be the largest in a much larger sample, only, perhaps, not that large as one would have hoped for. In that regard, it is not entirely true the magnitudes do not depend on the sample size. The magnitude *ranking* does not depend on the sample size, on the other hand, seems somewhat closer to the truth. The reason for this is using larger samples introduces a larger amount of variability of the relationship of interest into the sample and hence statistical calculus, which, in turn, *decreases* the difference between the groups thereby *decreasing* the magnitude of an effect.

* We shall touch the subject of *absolute* values more thoroughly later. One can likewise argue the magnitudes are rather stable yet the *calculus* of the magnitudes is flawed as it allows for such a great variability with increasing the sample size. This is probably the most correct way of looking at it, but it is far out of the scope of this booklet.

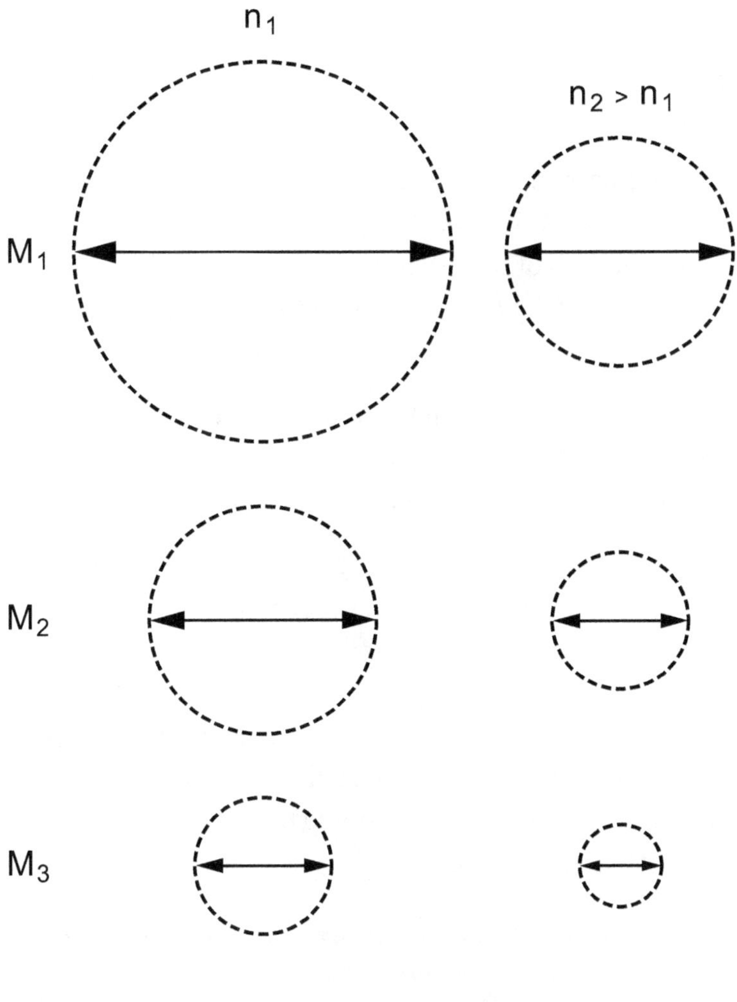

M_1, M_2, M_3........... magnitudes
n_1, n_2 ....sample sizes

Fig. 4. The magnitude ranking in the smaller (*left*) and larger (*right*) sample

In this small CT study, all frequentist statistics were calculated by hand, using a basic pocket calculator with four mathematical functions, and a square root button (Fig. 5).* In that regard, I would like to highlight certain points I find worth mentioning.

In ranking, both Wilcoxon and Spearman label the lowest value as rank 1, yet Wilcoxon does not whereas Spearman does consider the *sign* of the difference. This means, for example, for Wilcoxon – 5 equals + 5, whereas for Spearman – 5 is less than + 5!

In ranking, moreover, if the ranks are tied, both Wilcoxon and Spearman use the *mean* rank for each tie, whereas zero ranks in Wilcoxon are excluded from the calculus (n is *decreased*).

Although only statistically significant effects are considered true (that is to say, they did not appear by chance in the sample, and hence are true *outside* the sample, in the population), the size of an effect, the *magnitude*, was interpreted **regardless** of statistical significance as it represents ***the*** **most important** data of a scientific study. In fact, there are authors arguing only magnitudes with 95% CIs should be reported, and are voting against significance testing *altogether*, perhaps rightfully so.**

* For those interested, a 'CITIZEN SLD-100NR' was used. This was done deliberately to demonstrate the mathematical logic behind each statistical test, and to prove one does not need expensive statistical software to replicate the methodology of this small CT study.

** It is good to know with 95%CIs the overall error rate is indeed held to 5%, yet the same is not necessarily true with the standard $\alpha = .05$ level. For more on this, *see*, for example, Schmidt, 1996, p. 121.

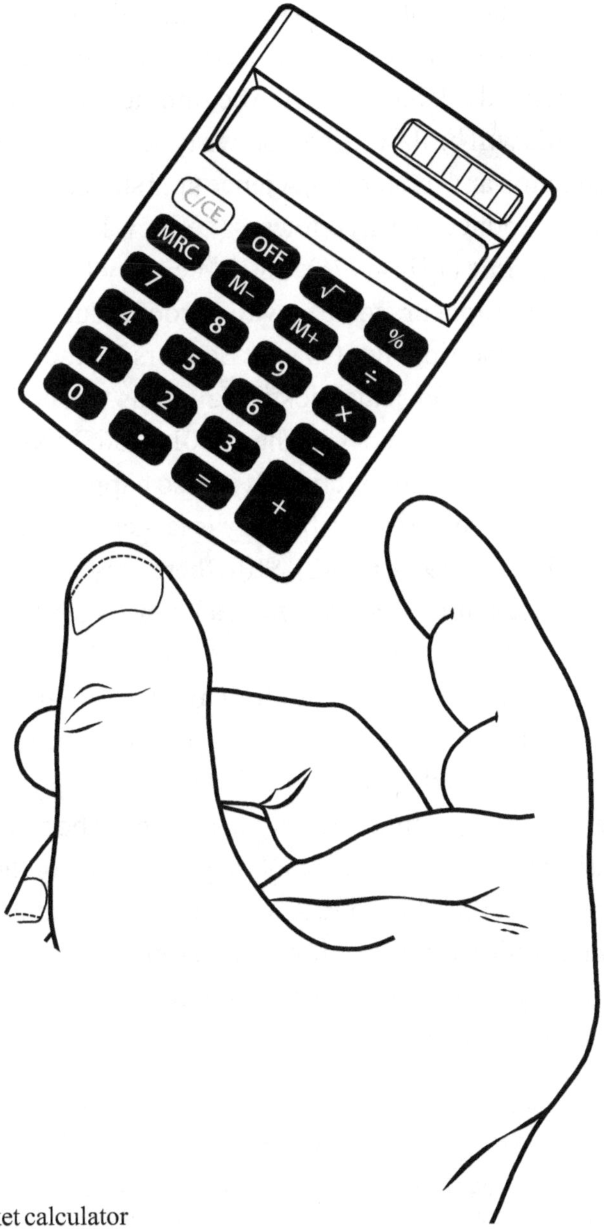

Fig. 5. Pocket calculator

The foundation of the house of science, though, is *logic*, not statistics—statistics is merely a *tool*. If your reasoning contains logical fallacies from the beginning, everything you do onwards will be flawed. Out of two types of logical reasoning (deduction and induction), science (and statistics) uses *induction* to produce new hypotheses (i.e., new knowledge). Since David Hume (1711–1776), an 18th century English philosopher, there appears to be no valid proof induction is a sound type of reasoning. For Charles Sanders Peirce (1839–1914), on the other hand, a diagnostic claim was 'abduction', a term Peirce 're-discovered' (Fischer, 2001, p. 365)*, yet a possible logical fallacy of deduction. It just so happens one needs to accept even scientific probability is far-fetched (Binder *et al.*, 2022; Popper, 1959, p. 142). Still, there exists a thing prior to logical reasoning—an *intuition*, a knowledge with no apparent foreknowledge. You 'feel' the truth *before* you rationalize it. On the basis of your clinical, and human experience (some may say, 'common sense'), you can intuitively 'feel' if something is right. This 'knowledge' may help you establish logical concepts that 'feel' right, and could be tested mathematically, using statistical tools to gain an aura of rational evidence through T-line of reasoning (Fig. 6).** Although induction is, indeed, flawed, nothing better has come up. Hence following T-line of reasoning, it seems a *valid clinical indicator* should meet *two logical concepts* to justify its practical use.

* How hard it was for Pearson himself to convince the sceptical medical community to use biostatistics, *see* Lu and Fang, 2003, pp. 9–10.

** Testing statistical hypotheses with no rhyme or reason means nothing but blurring the perspective without (more or less) solid logical background.

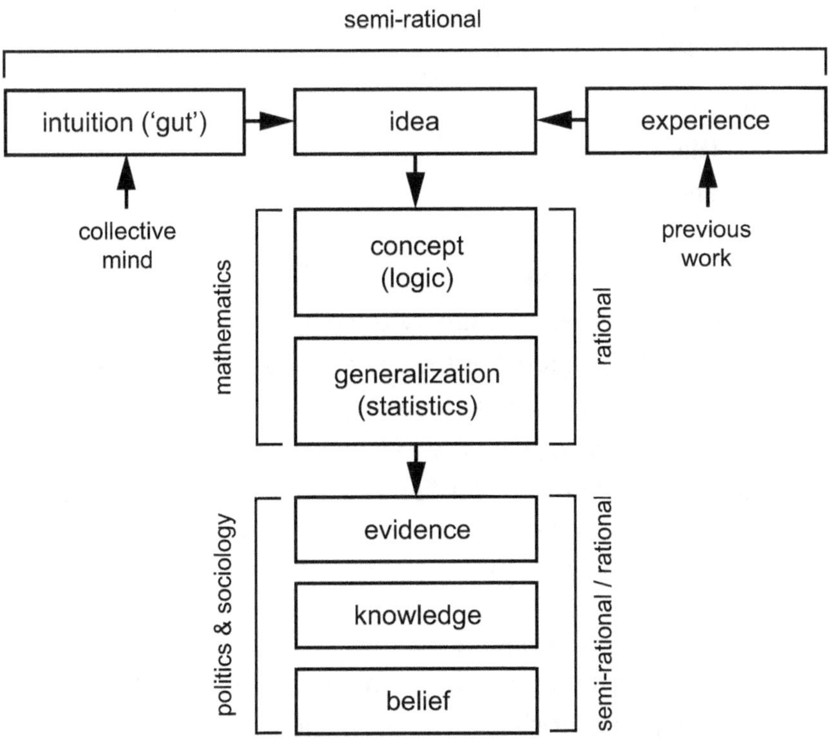

Fig. 6. T-line of reasoning

These logical concepts are:

i. *sorting* validity
(the indicator sorts out the condition, that is to say, the patient)

ii. *tracking* validity
(the indicator tracks therapeutic outcome, conservative and surgical alike).

These concepts stem from a simple understanding a physician needs to first recognize the patient, and then track the therapeutic outcome, either using conservative or surgical therapy. In other words: **the indicator must recognize, *trully* and *consistently*, who the patient is, and, also, whether or not the patient is doing *better* after therapy.** Therefore, a valid indicator should be of help with each step of the patient management (Fig. 7).*

This small CT study is not meant to give definite answers, but instead cast a light on a particular indicator, and suggest the path for its future investigation.

* It appears to me *any* indicator should satisfy these criteria, and not just the one investigated in this small CT study.

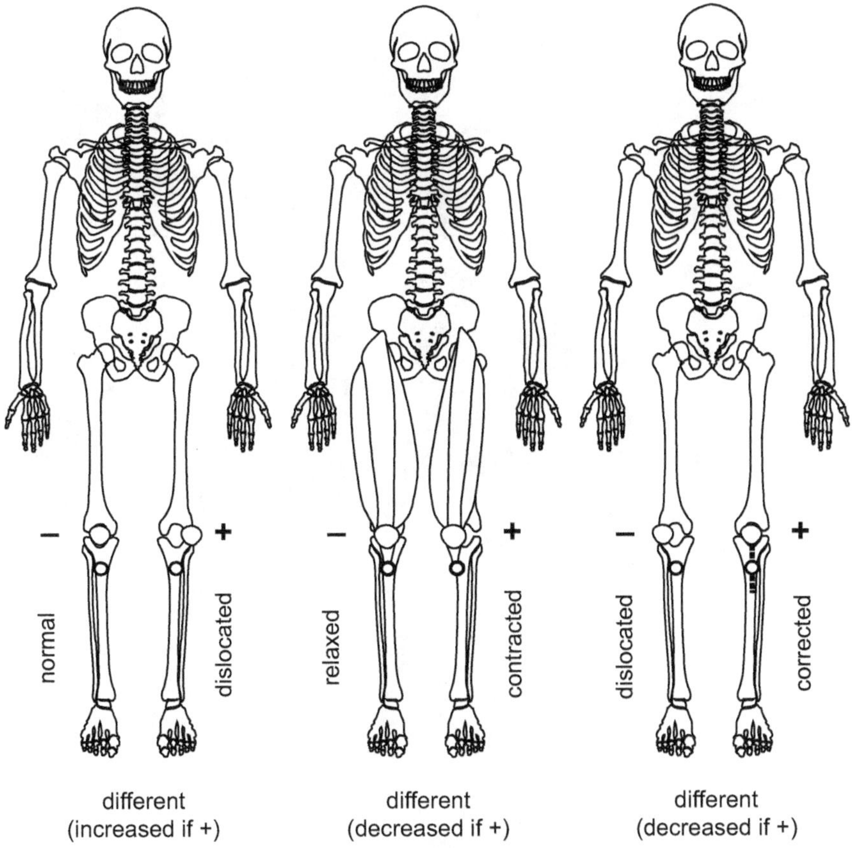

Fig. 7. Different logical concepts

2

2

Sorting Validity and External Confounders

To start a research, one should collect a *representative* sample, that is to say a sample in which the *variability* of the relationship of interest *equals* its variability in the population. After an idea is refined, the *magnitude* for the relationship of interest should be calculated. If the magnitude is *theoretical*, one should stop the research of the relationship of interest. If the magnitude is *practical*, however, one should test for *statistical significance* of the relationship of interest. If the relationship of interest *is* (statistically) *significant*, one should define the *cut-off* (a *threshold* between the negatives and the positives) and calculate *diagnostic validity*, namely *sensitivity* (a proportion of correctly detected *positives*), and *specificity* (a proportion of correctly detected *negatives*) (Altman, 1999, p. 410). If the relationship of interest is *not* (statistically) *significant*, one should collect a larger representative sample, and repeat the procedure. The algorithm is shown in Fig. 8. Bear in mind, however, the magnitude interpretation for a relationship of interest does not depend on the sample size whereas sensitivity and specificity do not depend on the *prevalence* (a proportion of *positives* in the sample), and thus, likewise, on the sample size (Altman, 1999, p. 411). Therefore, one needs to collect a *reasonable* sample size to start a new research. No firm consensus exists on the exact 'reasonable' size of a sample. In this small CT study, a sample of n = 15 sufficed.

I shall now consider an algorithm when a relationship of interest is an *indicator–condition* relationship.

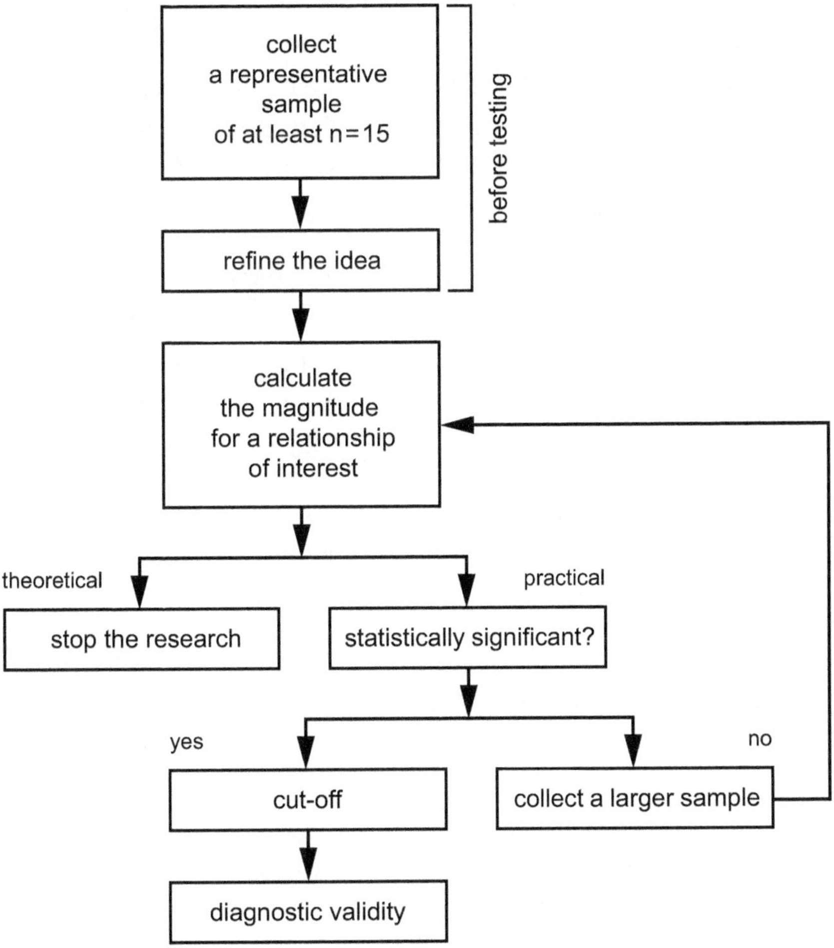

Fig. 8. Research algorithm of a scientific study

Yet, if one should compare the algorithm of a scientific study if the relationship of interest were the indicator–condition relationship, shown in Fig. 9, to the one previously explained, the only noticeable difference would be the *exclusion of confounders* during the refinement of an idea. This algorithmic step is **crucial** as it ensures the indicator–condition relationship is *exclusive.**

In the clinical setting, however, no firm consensus exists on the exact *percentage* the measures of diagnostic validity should meet other than a commonsensical rule of thumb: *the higher, the better.* For daily clinical practice, nevertheless, it appears sensitivity and specificity of at least 80% would suffice.**

This is, in a nutshell, what one needs to do in order to prove the indicator can classify the condition with 80% success rate to justify its practical use.

I shall now consider an indicator–condition relationship in the context of this small CT study.

* If one leaves be a possible confounder, one will never know to what extent it influences the indicator–condition relationship, and hence the classification ability of the indicator.

** In biological systems, a blood test, a clinical test or an imaging test with both sensitivity and specificity of at least 80% would be very difficult to design. Most of these tests incline to either one side of the diagnostic spectrum or the other. This is because variability is firmly rooted in biological environment. On that regard, having a balanced test with 80% success rate would be quite beneficial for daily clinical practice.

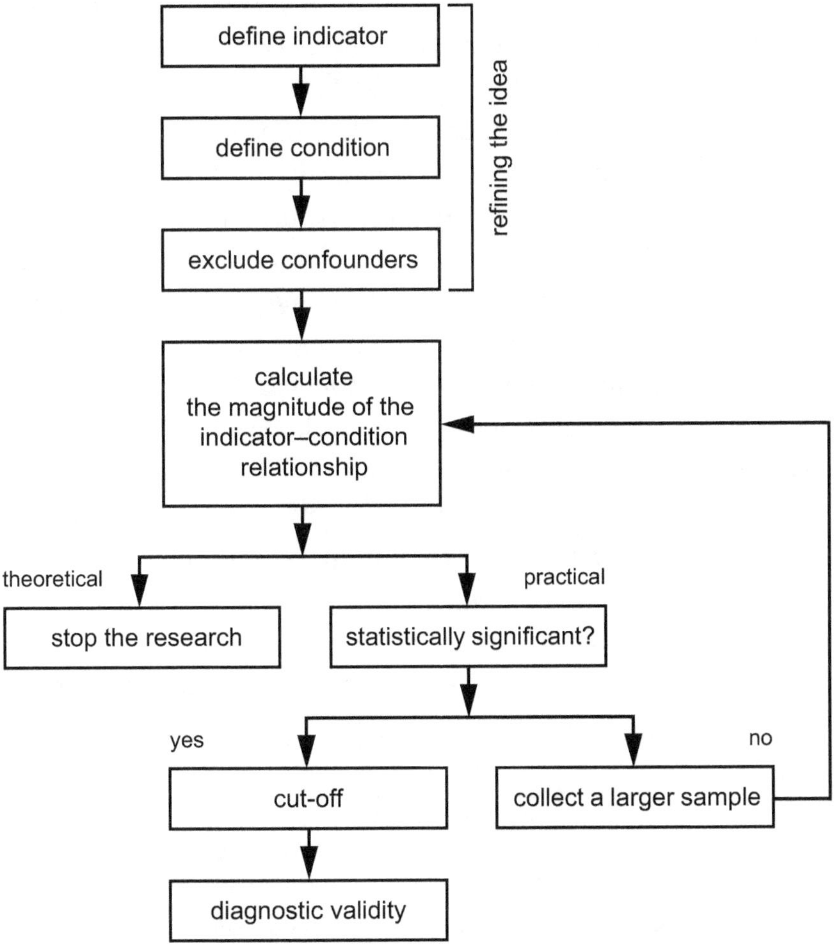

Fig. 9. Research algorithm of a scientific study if the relationship of interest were the indicator–condition relationship

An *indicator* is a variable that can indicate another variable, a *condition*. If an indicator changes *exclusively* with a condition, it *indicates* a condition.* In this small CT study, a study unit was a *knee*. An indicator was the *tibial tuberosity–tibial intercondylar midpoint* (TT-TIM) *distance*. A condition was the *recurrent* (two times or more) *patellar dislocation*. A negative (–) knee, a *negative*, was a knee without the condition ('normal' or a 'control'). A positive (+) knee, a *positive*, was a knee with the condition ('abnormal' or a 'case'). If you want to test an indicator's sorting validity, both negatives, and positives should have the *same* anatomy (hence it would be ideal if they belonged to a *natural pair*, that is to say—the *same* participant), as well as intact skin and subcutaneous tissue, bones, muscles, tendons, ligaments, and the intracapsular part of the knee (hence an indicator can indicate the only thing different between them, a patellar dislocation, the condition) whereas their confounders should be *excluded* (hence the indicator–condition relationship is exclusive) (Fig.10).** Given that an indicator was a *numerical* variable, its value should have *increased* when the condition was present.***

* The English verb *indicate* comes from the Latin verb *indicāre*: *declare, mention*, formed by the prefix *in-* and the verb *dicāre*: *proclaim* (Hoad, 1996, p. 233). Therefore, the indicator *proclaims* the condition (if present).

** Although this sounds reasonable, it is very difficult to collect suitable negatives, more so with natural pairs, especially in retrospective research. Due to practical reasons, one should at least try to exclude the most common confounders.

*** This is because a condition is perceived as an (unwanted) *gain* (one 'got' the disease).

–/+ ......condition (recurrent patellar dislocation)
c....... confounder
I.............indicator

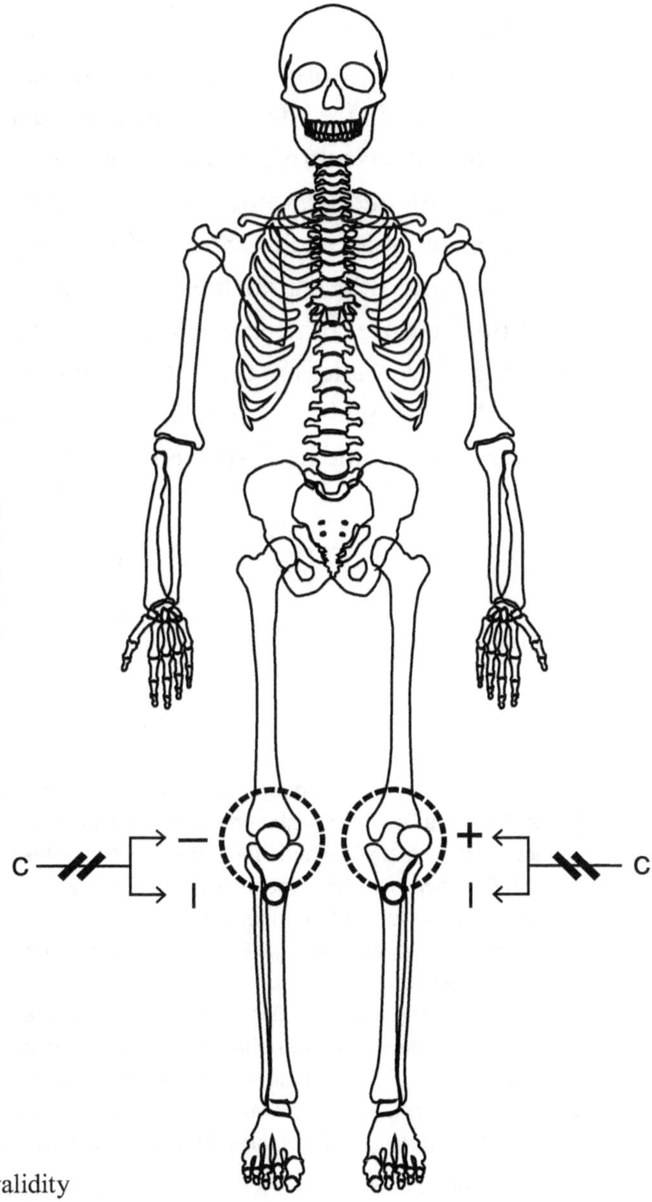

Fig. 10. Sorting validity

Using natural pairs means the participants were *independent* to each other whereas their knees were *dependent* to each other (because two knees forming a pair belonged to the *same* participant) (Fig. 11). Paired design is an *advantage* of orthopedic research. What is more, it is an easy way of excluding many external confounders, some of them, possibly, *unknown*. For example, variables such as body height, body weight, pelvic diameters and alike cannot have a confounding effect on the condition because both knees belonged to the *same* participant and thus the variables are the same in both negatives and positives.* In this small CT study, the simplest of paired designs was used, that could be described by a *square diagonal matrix*: **

$$d(a_{11}, a_{22}, \dots, a_{nn}) = \begin{bmatrix} a_{11} & 0 \cdots 0 \\ 0 & a_{22} \cdots 0 \\ \vdots & \vdots \ddots \vdots \\ 0 & 0 \cdots a_{nn} \end{bmatrix}.$$

* A common misconception about the design of this kind of a study is that if one studies an indicator on knees from *different* individuals, it would suffice to use a statistical test for *independent* samples, and the problem is solved. This is not true because the statistical test will find the difference (if it existed), yet cannot tell its cause. Imagine a negative from an individual A, and a positive from an individual B. Let us say the indicator was significantly different. However, the individual A is a man of 180 cm in height, and weighs 75 kg whereas the individual B is a man of 201 cm in height and weighs 125 kg. That alone (and who knows what else) might represent external confounding to the values of the indicator or the condition one has no way to exclude or even know about. In other words: the *difference found may be a result of external confounding*, and not the indicator–condition relationship.

** For more on this, *see*, for example, Lu and Fang, 2003, pp. 57–9.

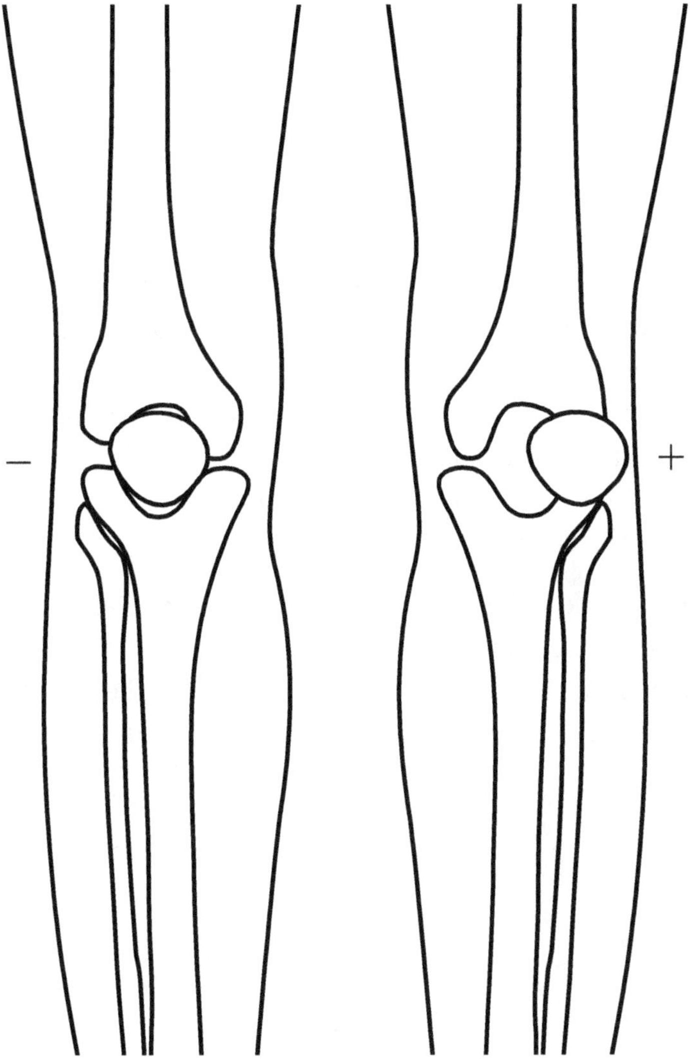

Fig. 11. Natural (knee) pair

In *positives*, the orthopedic charts were retrospectively reviewed, and two or more patellar dislocations were reported. In fact, **87% (13/15)** of the positives had **more than two** patellar dislocations, which is in keeping with recent stringent criteria of the *Lyonnaise School of Orthopedics* defining the recurrent patellar instability as that with **three or more** patellar dislocations.

What follows is a table of 15 anonymized patients included in this small CT study, along with orthopedic clinical remarks. It is, in fact, a pilot sample I used to later undertake a much larger study published in the highly esteemed scientific journal *International Orthopaedics* (SICOT) in 2021.*

* The original idea of TT-TIM distance is a bit older—as much as I can recall, it dates into the year 2011.

Inidividual	Total patellar dislocations	
	Left knee	*Right knee*
1	—	multiple (3)
2	multiple	—
3	—	multiple (4)
4	multiple (at least 2)	—
5	multiple	—
6	—	multiple
7	multiple	—
8	multiple (6)	—
9	multiple (at least 2)	—
10	—	multiple (4–5)
11	—	multiple (7)
12	—	multiple (4)
13	multiple	—
14	multiple (4)	—
15	multiple	—

n	Sex	Age	Date of CT screening	mA		kV		Major orthopedic remarks
				Q relaxation	*Q contraction*	*Q relaxation*	*Q contraction*	
1	M	15	2015-09-14	47	52	130	130	(R) multiple patellar dislocations (3), CT confirmed intra-articular loose body of 10 mm in diameter in the suprapatellar reccess due to recurrent patellar dislocations, no fracture or effusion, clinically unstable patella, positive Turner sign
2	F	15	2014-04-18	51	52	130	130	(L) multiple patellar dislocations without trauma, especially after running, a hypermobile patella, negative test for menisci, mild quadriceps muscle hypotrophy, ligaments intact
3	F	16	2014-01-08	49	51	130	130	(R) multiple patellar dislocations (4), a small fragment
4	M	17	2014-04-04	45	45	130	130	(L) multiple patellar dislocations (at least two)
5	F	22	2015-02-03	47	52	130	130	(L) first of multiple patellar dislocation appeared while walking, CT confirmed a small subchondral cyst of 3 mm in diameter in the medial condyle of the tibia
6	F	15	2014-06-06	51	42	130	130	(R) first of multiple patellar dislocations appeared while dancing
7	F	29	2014-12-23	55	55	130	130	(L) multiple patellar dislocations, maltracking, negative test for menisci, habitual patellar dislocations
8	F	23	2013-07-31	48	44	130	130	(L) multiple patellar dislocations (6), parapatellar cramps, pain, positive J sign, luxabile patella, femoral trochlear dysplasia, a small calcification of 5 mm in diameter at the enthesis of the medial retinaculum

n	Sex	Age	Date of CT screening	mA		kV		Major orthopedic remarks
				Q relaxation	*Q contraction*	*Q relaxation*	*Q contraction*	
9	M	22	2014-11-11	100	100	130	130	(L) multiple patellar dislocations (at least two)
10	F	14	2014-09-16	45	50	130	130	(R) multiple patellar dislocations (4–5), hypotrophy of the quadriceps muscle, positive Turner sign, no effusion or swelling, open growth plates
11	M	17	2015-10-21	99	117	130	130	(R) multiple patellar dislocations (7), positive Turner sign, clinically unstable patella
12	M	24	2015-01-20	48	50*	130	130*	(R) first of multiple patellar dislocations (4) appeard while playing football, no effusion, positive Turner sign (++/+++), positive apprehension test, full range of motion, dysplastic patella (Wiberg IV)
13	F	33	2014-07-18	40	49	130	130	(L) multiple patellar dislocations, pain, positive apprehension test, cortical dysplasia of the tibia, possibly NOF or osteoid osteoma
14	F	18	2014-02-19	49	51	130	130	(L) multiple patellar dislocations (4)
15	M	18	2014-07-09	49	52	130	130	(L) multiple patellar dislocations, CT confirmed intra-articular loose body of 13 mm in diameter adjacent to the lateral femoral condyle, with a small effusion due to recurrent patellar dislocations

* 5 mm cut thickness; CT, computed tomography; F, female; L, left knee; M, male; n, sample size; Q, quadriceps muscle; R, right knee. **Note:** Given that the author knew the full identity of participants, during statistical analysis they have been ranked according to their last names in *descending* order, from A to Z, and not according to the date of CT screening.

A horizontal hypothetical antecedent of bilaterally symmetric animals had two poles, and a horizontal line of symmetry (Matoničkin and Erben, 1994, p. 52). Following verticalization, the human line of symmetry became what we now call the *vertical* (body) *line of symmetry* (*axis*). A leg, as a separate part of the human body, had its own vertical line of symmetry, the *mechanical axis of the leg* (MAL), connecting the relative middles of the hip and the ankle while passing through the relative middle of the knee, or slightly *medial* (Paley, 2002, p. 12). In healthy individuals, the quadriceps mechanism is in the MAL, and, especially, its insertion (He *et al.*, 2013, p. 502).* Should the quadriceps insertion become too distant from the absolute middle of the leg, that is the MAL, mostly to the *outer* side, the lateral forces acting upon the knee would increase and perpetually dislocate the patella, causing *recurrent patellar instability*. Therefore, an indicator of the condition should be a distance between the point reflecting the quadriceps mechanism insertion (the tibial tuberosity), and the point reflecting the absolute middle of the leg, the MAL in the frontal plane. The problem is the absolute middle of the leg is *unknown*. Instead, one could use a handful of its *relative* middles (Moreland *et al.*, 1987, p. 746). The indicator in this small CT study uses a *new* point, the *tibial intercondylar midpoint* (TIM) at the proximal part of the tibia, and is therefore called the *tibial tuberosity–tibial intercondylar midpoint* (TT-TIM) *distance*. It is expressed in *millimeters*, as a *positive integer*. Moreland's points reflecting relative middles of the leg as well as TIM are shown in Fig. 12.

* In healthy individuals, the middle of the medial and middle third of the tibial tuberosity is maximally 5.38 mm from the tibial mechanical axis.

a........ midpoint of the femoral notch ('Roman arch')
b........ midpoint of the tibial spines
c........ midpoint of the femoral condyles
d........ midpoint of the soft tissue
e......midpoint of the tibia
f........ tibial intercondylar midpoint (new point)

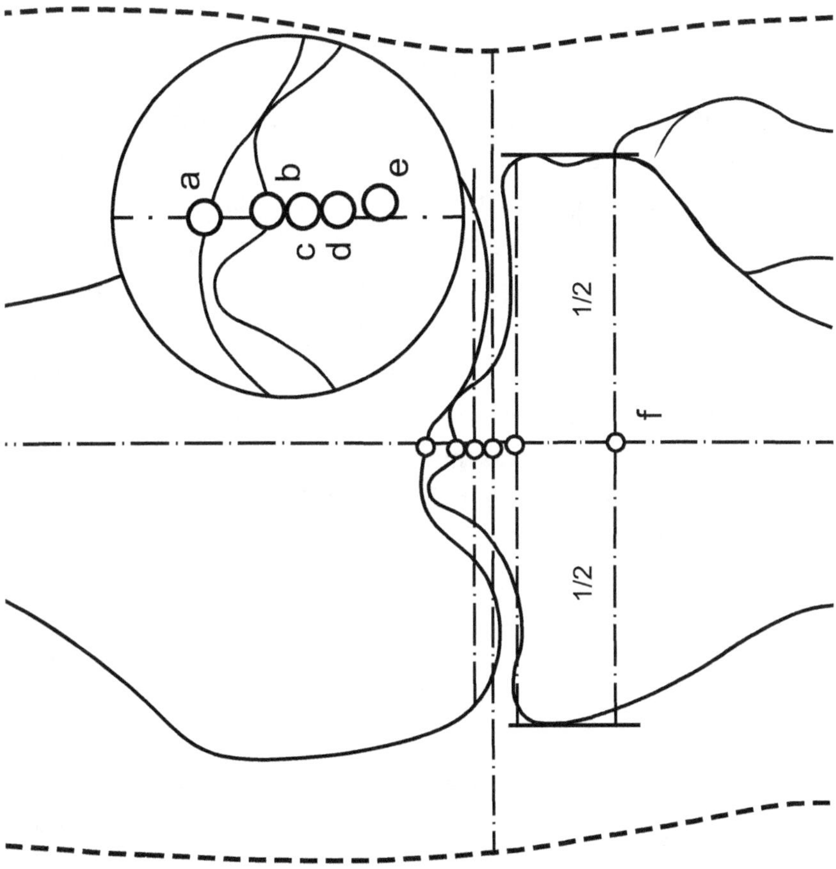

Fig. 12. Moreland's points and the new point (**f**) reflecting the relative middles of the leg/knee

An attentive reader might have been puzzled by the absolute and relative middles. In theory, there is only *one* middle of an object, and that is the *absolute* ('true') *middle.** If one likens the vertical line of symmetry of a leg to the MAL, and they are primordially conceptualized as such, they both pass vertically through the absolute middle of the leg, and, thus, the absolute middle of the knee. The absolute middle of the knee has, therefore, two features: 1) it is *unknown* (hence *invisible*), and 2) it is *always* in the middle (hence *static*). For didactical purposes, one can imagine a 'true' middle of a knee as an *invisible wall* in the frontal plane (Fig. 13). Because one does not know the coordinates of the absolute middle, different middles have been used *relative* to different anatomical structures (this is why the middle of the hip is relative to the midpoint of the femoral head, the middle of the knee is relative to various points such as the midpoint of the 'Roman arch' or the intercondylar midpoint of the proximal part of the tibia, and so on). This brings one to an inevitable conclusion: one will **never** know the 'true' middle of the leg/knee because not only one cannot know whether the relative middle reflects the 'true' middle, but one cannot even investigate it since the 'true' middle is not available for comparison (and if it were, of course, one would not need a relative middle of the leg/knee to begin with).

* Take, for example, the temperature scales. The Celsius (C) temperature scale is *relative*, that is to say it relates to a *particular* substance, the *water* (for example, when water freezes, it is 0° C, when it boils, it is 100° C) whereas Kelvin temperature scale is *absolute,* that is to say it relates to *any* substance. This is why 0° Kelvin is called an 'absolute 0'. The absolute 0 is not yet proven, but physicists have come extremely close to it, proving 1° Kelvin in some distant cosmic nebula. Remember we even relate time to space!

?.......absolute middle of the leg/knee (an invisible and static wall)

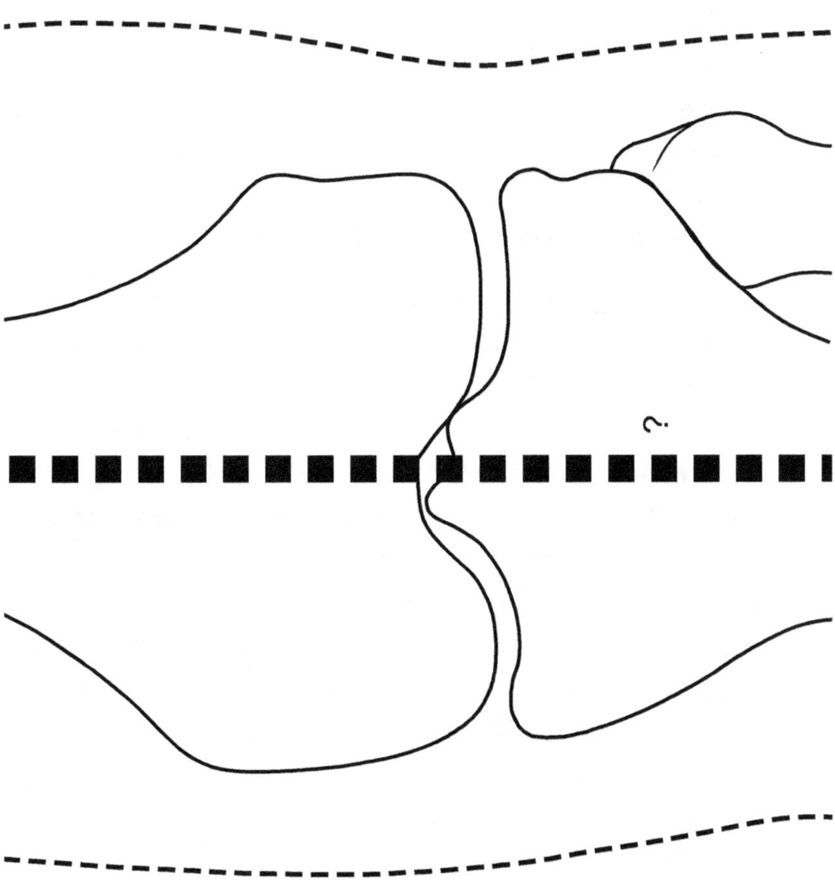

Fig. 13. Absolute middle of the leg/knee

Why is this 'riddle of the middle' so important? It is, actually, of utmost importance because the main objective of this small CT study was to design an indicator of the condition as a distance between the point reflecting the quadriceps mechanism insertion, the tibial tuberosity (TT), and the point reflecting the 'true' middle of the leg/knee/the MAL in the frontal plane. If one does not know where to find the'true' middle, one cannot find the 'true' distance as well as trust any of the relative middles to represent a 'true' middle of the knee. Since the distance itself *is* the indicator, this makes the design of the 'true' indicator of the condition **impossible**. The best one can do is to accept the fact one shall never know whether or not the relative middle reflects the 'true' middle of the knee. Fortunately, however, this may not be an issue in daily clinical practice.

The 'true' middle is an invisible wall: *invisible* and *static*. This means a point reflecting a relative middle of the knee should be *visible* and *static*. Even if one cannot test whether or not a relative middle reflects the 'true' middle of the knee, one can still test whether or not it is *static*. In daily clinical practice, this means TIM should always be in the exact bone spot (the middle) of the proximal part of the tibia from one bone to another, from one individual to another. The tibial tuberosity, however, is the insertion of the dynamic quadriceps mechanism. Hence, in this small CT study, the indicator was a distance between two points: *one, visible and static* (*TIM*), *and the other, visible and dynamic* (*TT*). If one imagined the former as a *wall*, and the latter as a *ball*, one could call it the **'wall and ball theory'** (Fig. 14).

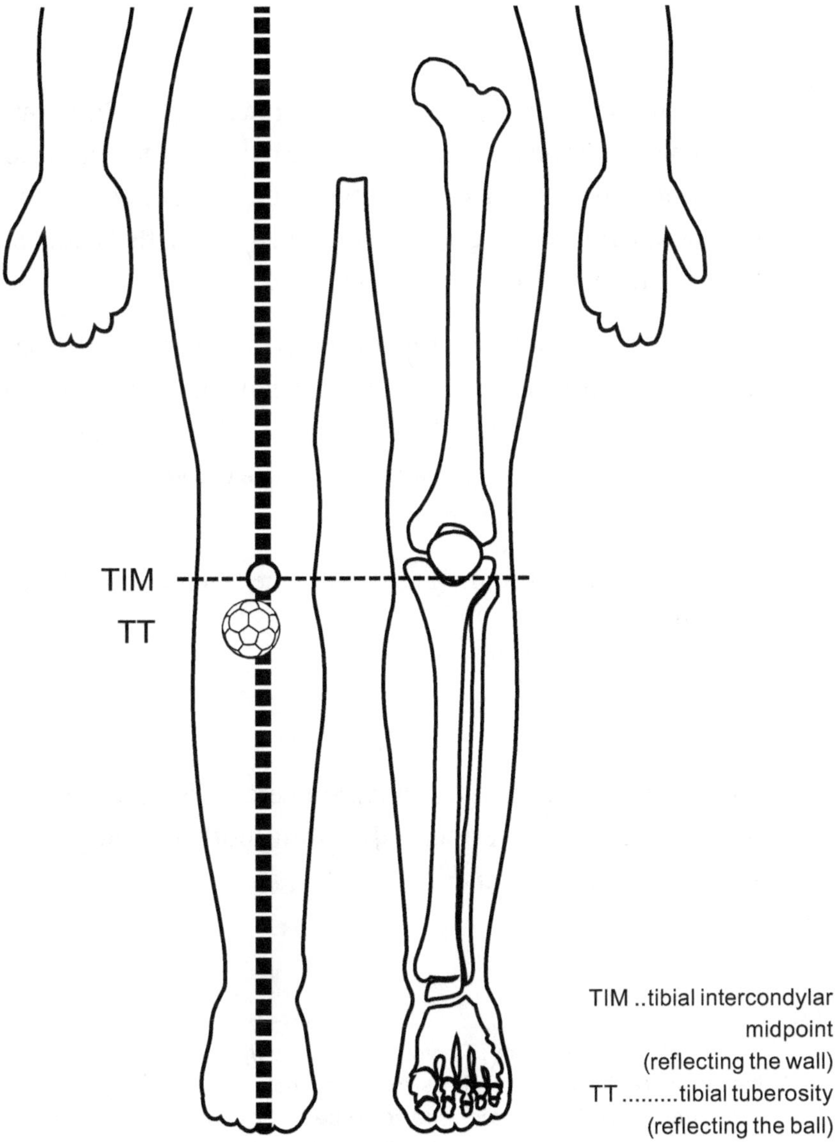

Fig. 14. Wall and ball theory

If the wall were a *static* point, and the ball were a *dynamic* point, then it would be obvious to assume the ball going towards the wall would make the distance between them *decrease*. On the contrary, with the ball going away from the wall, the distance between them would *increase* (Fig. 15).

Therefore, an action bringing the ball closer to the wall, that is to say, bringing the quadriceps mechanism insertion (TT) closer to the relative middle of the knee (TIM), and that is the **quadriceps contraction**, should *decrease* the value of the indicator (TT-TIM distance).

This simple understanding represents the essence of the 'wall and ball theory'.

It is now clear TIM should be a *static* whereas TT is a *dynamic** point in the pair. Nevertheless, defining both of these points should be *standardized*.

* In describing the TT point, an adjective *dynamic* was used rather than *variable*. The anatomical position of both points, that is to say the *position of the point relative to the bone*, **must be static** (stable, unchangeable). The adjective *dynamic* refers not to the variable anatomical position but to the variable *spatial position of a bone with the TT point on it*. On the contrary, the TG point (*see* further) varies considerably in its anatomical (bone) position.

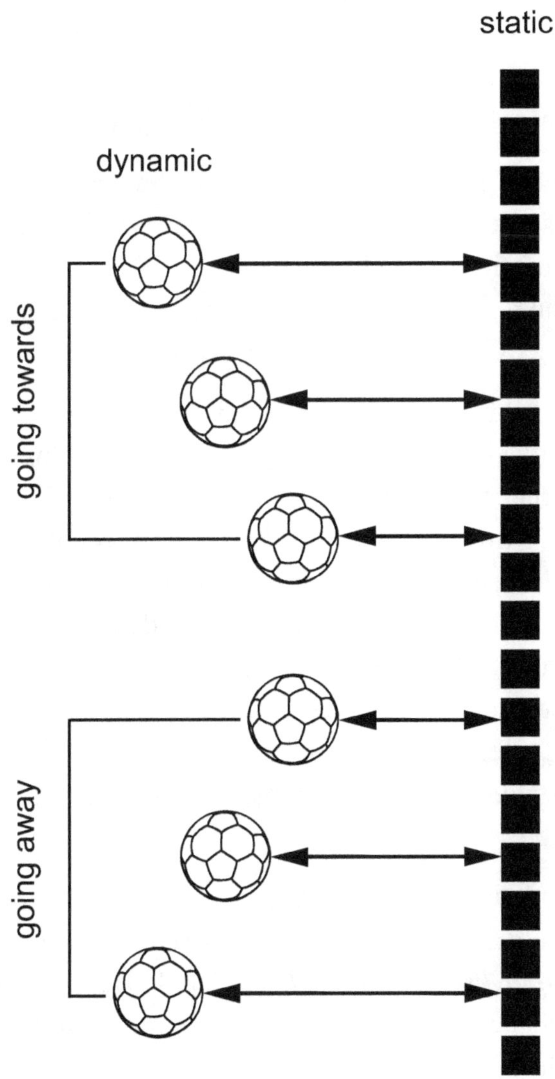

Fig. 15. The essence of the 'wall and ball theory'

The first aspect of the indicator standardization is one needs to ensure that the midpoint of the proximal part of the tibia is always defined *at the same anatomical level of the bone.* To this aim, the reference CT image should be quick and easy to find.

During CT scrolling in caudo-cranial direction, the fibular head was used as a *guide*. Therefore, the first CT image where the top of the fibular head was no longer visible (the ‘headless cut’) was the *reference* CT image. The procedure of choosing the reference CT image is shown in Fig. 16.

Since the top of the fibular head is mostly located at the same anatomical level from one leg to another, from one individual to another, this makes it a suitable guide in choosing the reference CT image to define TIM position. What is more, even if, for whatever reason, this procedure was not achievable (for example, there was no fibula), one could calculate the millimeter level at which the top of the fibular head would have been located had the fibula been present. This would make the use of this reference level applicable in scientific fields such as *anthropology*, where, perhaps, only the tibia might have been available.

The arthritic changes of the proximal tibiofibular joint are relatively rare and occur mostly as a complication of *ankylosing spondylitis* (Canna *et al.*, 2013, p. 1). Hence, there is a very little chance fibular head arthrosis could meaningfully affect the selection of the ‘headless cut’.

In this small CT study, in all thirty legs, the ‘headless cut’ was quick and easy to find.

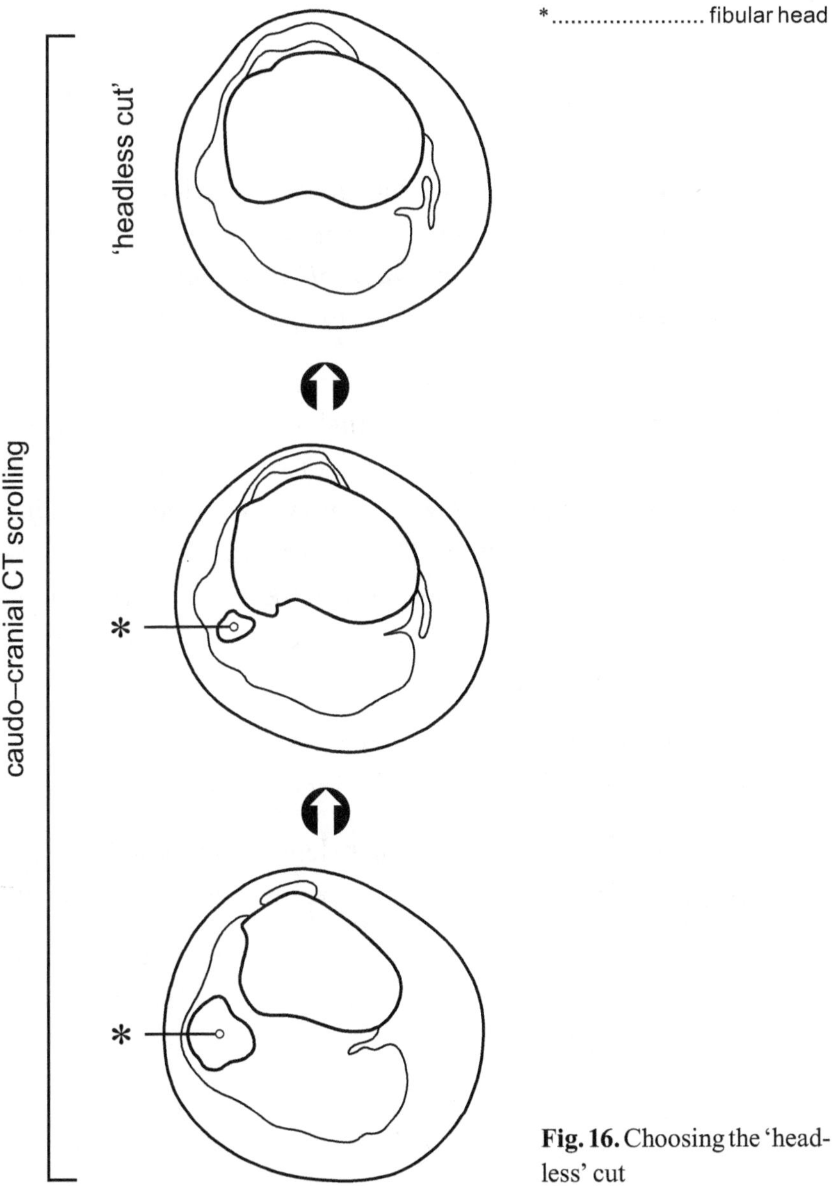

Fig. 16. Choosing the 'headless' cut

The second aspect of the indicator standardization is one needs to ensure that the midpoint of the proximal part of the tibia is always defined *in the same anatomical position on the bone.* To this end, the *pericondylar rectangle* was drawn (Fig. 17).

With the use of a pericondylar rectangle rather than a circle geometrical approximation of the midpoint becomes much more convenient. One needs to draw two internal diagonals in the pericondylar rectangle, and then a vertical midline passing through their intersection. This vertical midline in the transverse plane represents a midpoint of the proximal part of the tibia in the frontal plane. The next step would be to copy the vertical midline on all CT images of the series.

The pericondylar rectangle might be especially valuable in preventing misclassification of individual borderline cases.

In this small CT study, in all thirty legs, the pericondylar rectangle and the vertical midline were quick and easy to draw.

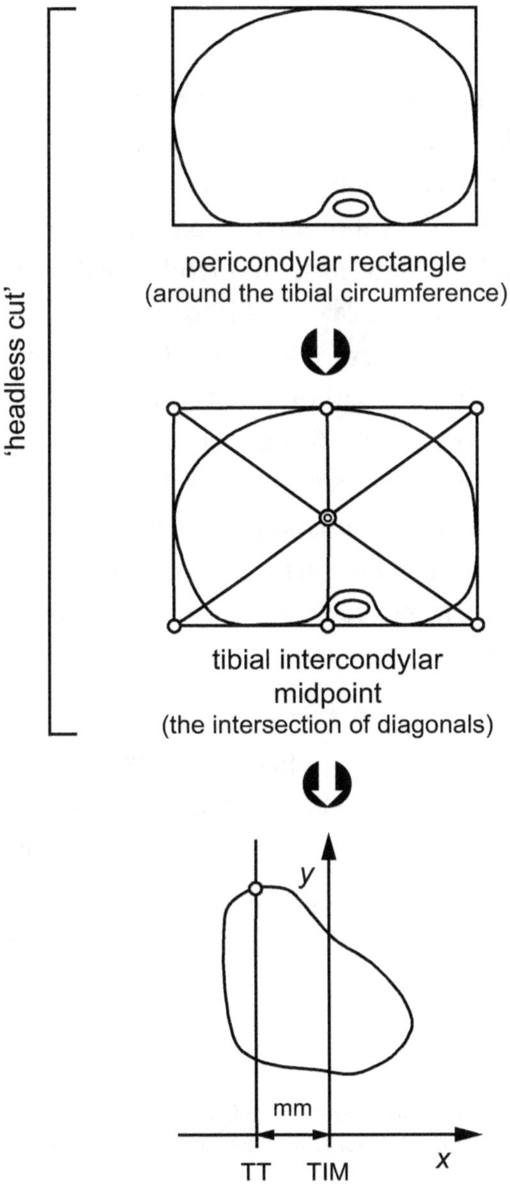

mm....................millimeters
TT................tibial tuberosity
TIM ....tibial intercondylar midpoint
x,*y*................................ axes (of the orthogonal coordinate system)

Fig. 17. Tibial intercondylar midpoint constructed using a pericondylar rectangle on the 'headless' cut

Enclosing the circumference of the tibial figure in the transverse plane by a pericondylar rectangle may be regarded as a reflection of 'Gestalt' theory of human perception, defined a century ago by German psychologists Max Wertheimer (1880–1943), Kurt Koffka (1886–1941) and Wolfgang Köhler (1887–1967) (Al-Alwan, Al-Bazzaz and Ali, 2022, p. 3). This suddenly becomes more evident when the tibial circumference is *incomplete* due to a pathological condition (Fig. 18). The incomplete tibial circumference results in the *incomplete* pericondylar rectangle. Nevertheless, following the principle of *closure* (*rectification*), one of the main laws of 'Gestalt' theory, the incomplete form is perceived (as well as reconstructed) as *complete*, hence the measurement is possible even in these disadvantageous circumstances.*

Considering a rectangle is a simple figure, stable, regular, continuous, and a unified form, one might regard this configuration as 'good' with providing consistency in perception of different tibiae. It certainly contributes to the *Prägnanz* ('precision') of the whole.

* One might notice it is rather easy to visually estimate the central focal point of a rectangle, so it seems books, windows and screens are not rectangular by chance.

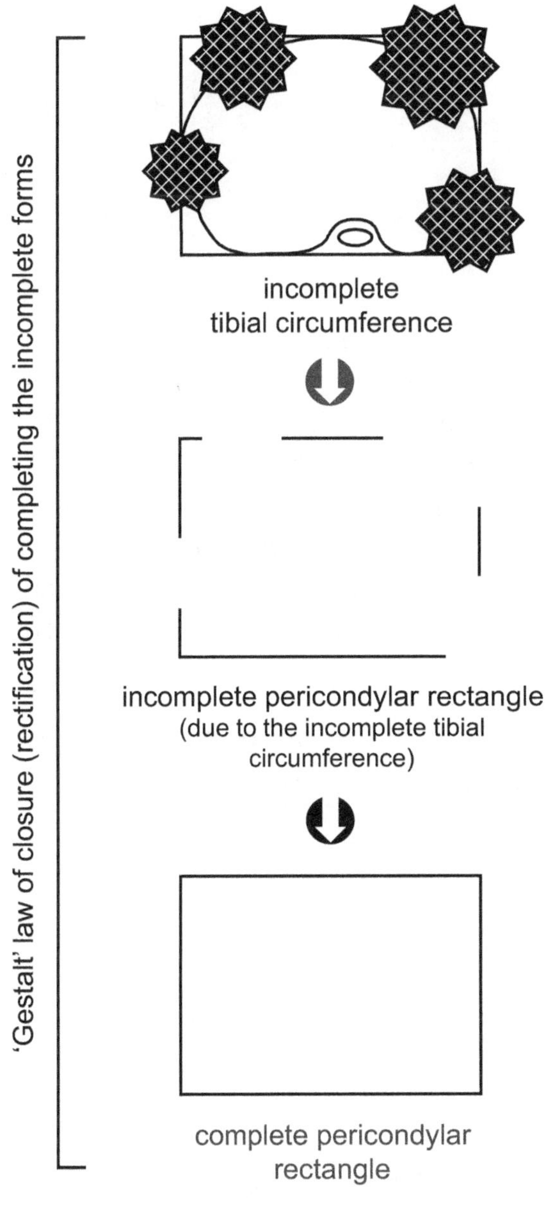

Fig. 18. 'Gestalt' closure of the incomplete tibial circumference with the pericondylar rectangle

The *Prägnanz* ('precision') of the whole principle may appear somewhat aetherical and a bit vague, yet, in fact, it is a purely practical feature of the TT-TIM distance design, ensuring its *robustness*. Thanks to this principle, one is able to measure the TT-TIM distance in various conditions *before* and *after* surgical procedures and mostly with regard to any other condition dealing with the circumference of the proximal part of the tibia.

The important practical value of the principle on real 'headless CT cuts' of three individuals is shown in Fig. 19.

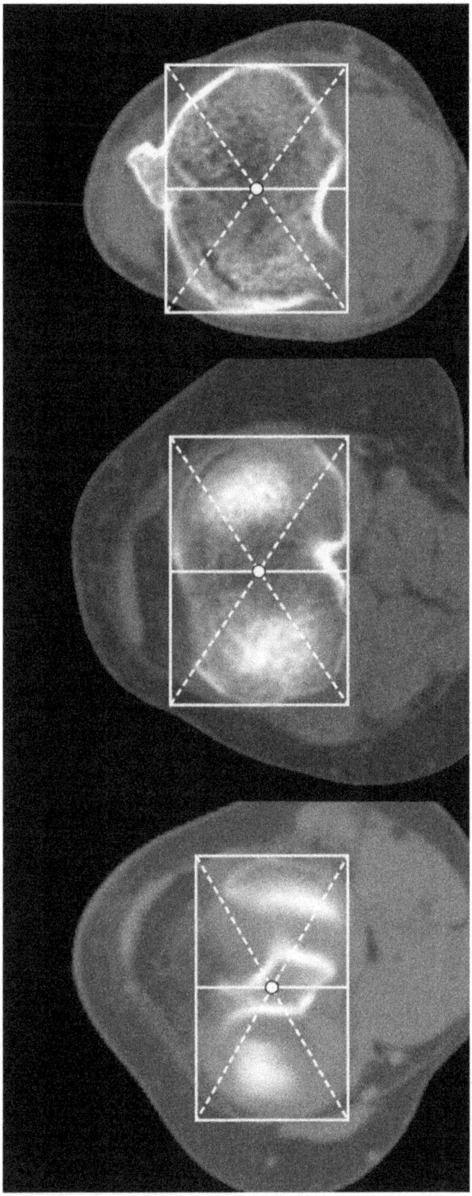

Fig. 19. 'Gestalt'closure of the incomplete tibial circumference with the pericondylar rectangle ('headless CT cuts' of three individuals, locating the TIM)

The third aspect of indicator standardization is one needs to ensure that the midpoint of the top of the tibial tuberosity is always defined *at the same anatomical level of the bone*. This actually goes for all the indicators in the field, as they *all* use this reference point as a landmark of quadriceps mechanism insertion. To this aim, the reference CT image should be quick and easy to find.

During CT scrolling in cranio-caudal direction, the CT image where the tibial tuberosity was the most prominent, that is to say the most *anterior* (the 'prominent cut') was the *reference* CT image (Fig. 20).*

In this small CT study, in all thirty legs, the 'prominent cut' was quick and easy to find.

* I do not think a selection of a slightly different neighbouring level, for example that where the lower part of the quadriceps tendon was in contact with the bony insertion would have a substantial impact on the measurement of the indicator, at least with integer values, although it may be a matter for future investigation.

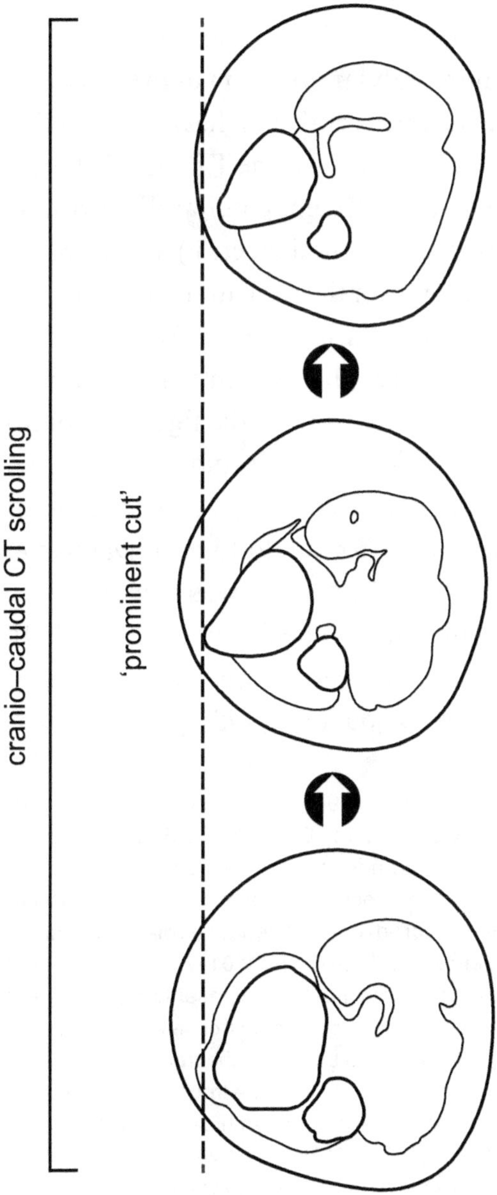

Fig.20. Choosing the 'prominent cut'

Therefore, in this small CT study, the indicator was the millimeter distance between the relative middle of the knee, reflected by the tibial intercondylar midpoint of the proximal part of the tibia on the 'headless cut', and the midpoint of tibial tuberosity on the 'prominent cut', the TT-TIM distance, whereas the condition was recurrent patellar dislocations (two or more). Interestingly, in their pioneering work, written in French, the original authors of the measurement used *central X-ray* (*XR*) *beam* to define the middle of the leg/the knee/the MAL. Although it was not explicitly mentioned, it is obvious from the context, and more so from the figures (Goutallier *et al.*, 1978, p. 424: 'TA-GT'). In their study, however, the femoral trochlea had a *regular* shape (Fig. 21). Though used on XR with normative values from 10 to 15 mm (Dahhan *et al.*, 1981, pp. 36–7, Fig. 11.D), the method was quickly transferred to CT, yet without validity check (Judet *et al.*, 1979). From 1987, with the use of two superimposed reference images, it became wider known (Dejour *et al.*, 1987, p. 39: Fig. 9).*

* Even though Folke Knutsson (1901–1993), a well-known Swedish radiologist, introduced the German term 'Dysplasie' in 1940s (Knutsson, 1941, p. 375), the original French authors *did not consider it*. In their measurement, they surmised the femoral trochlea had a *regular* shape. If it were indeed regular, the bottom of its groove *would* reflect a relative middle of the femur, that is to say, the knee (Nizić, 2012, pp. 1101–2). Yet, this created a certain confusion in years to come as most of the patients with recurrent patellar instability have an *irregular* shape of femoral trochlea. It significantly decreased the practical usefulness of the bottom of the trochlear groove as the point reflecting the relative middle of the knee (the trochlear groove or TG point). Due to dysplastic changes of the femoral trochlea, the TG point may be very difficult to define (Nizić, 2013, p. NP53). The variable shape of the femoral trochlea makes the position of the TG point variable (= dynamic).

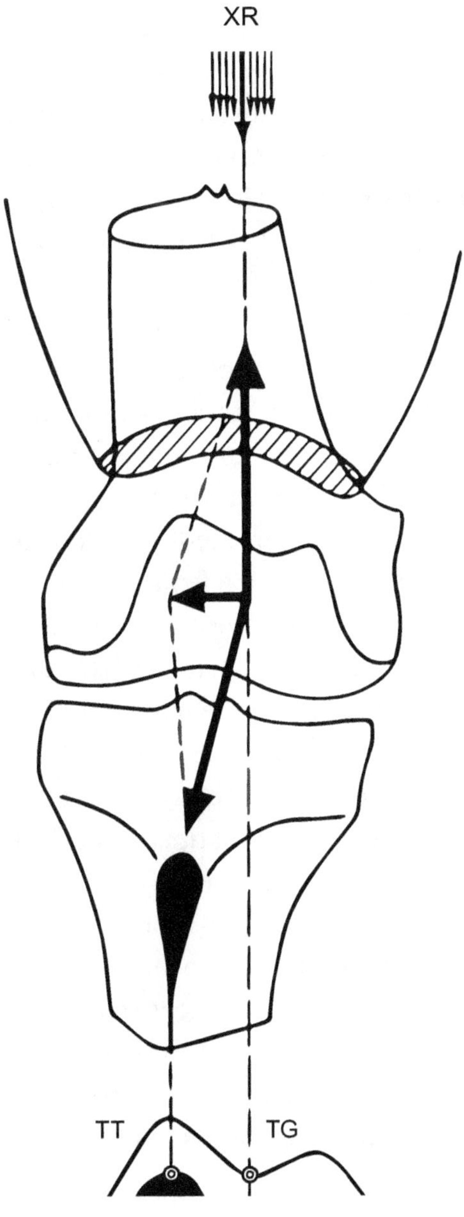

TG...........(femoral) trochlear groove (point) (the relative middle of the knee)
TT................tibial tuberosity
XR...............................X-rays

Fig. 21. Trochlear groove (TG) point (implied to reflect a relative middle of the knee)

(from the original paper of Goutallier, Bernageau and Lecudonnec, 1978, p. 424, Fig. 1)

Namely, the anatomical (bony) position of TG point, and thus TT-TG distance, is a *function* of femoral trochlear dysplasia (FTD). FTD occurs in 70–90% of positives. Hence, FTD and positives occur *in tandem*. Since TT-TG distance is a function of FTD, it likewise, *indirectly*, recognizes positives. TT-TG is, therefore, an **indirect indicator of positives**. However, in daily clinical practice, one knows already whether a knee is a positive. What one *really* wants is to track a therapeutic outcome, conservative and surgical alike. TT-TG distance cannot do this because its TG point *is not static*. To understand this, imagine, on the contrary, TT point were static instead of dynamic (Fig. 22). Now, if femoral trochlea were *regular*, the anatomical (bony) position of its TG point would be static (on the same spot from one femur to another), repeatedly resulting in *equal* TT-TG distances. On the other hand, if femoral trochlea were *irregular*, which is true in most positives, the anatomical (bony) position of its TG point would be a function of FTD, and thus not static (not on the same spot from one femur to another), repeatedly (and erroneously) resulting in *different* TT-TG distances. In comparison, the anatomical (bony) position of TIM point is static (on the same spot from one tibia to another), repeatedly resulting in *equal* TT-TIM distances. If one wants to track a therapeutic outcome, the anatomical (bony) position of the point reflecting the relative middle of the knee **must be static**. So, TT-TIM can, and TT-TG cannot detect a change in spatial position of TT point, which is crucial if one wants to track a therapeutic outcome. Ironically, the same thing, FTD, enabling the TT-TG distance to recognize a positive, prevents it from tracking a therapeutic outcome.

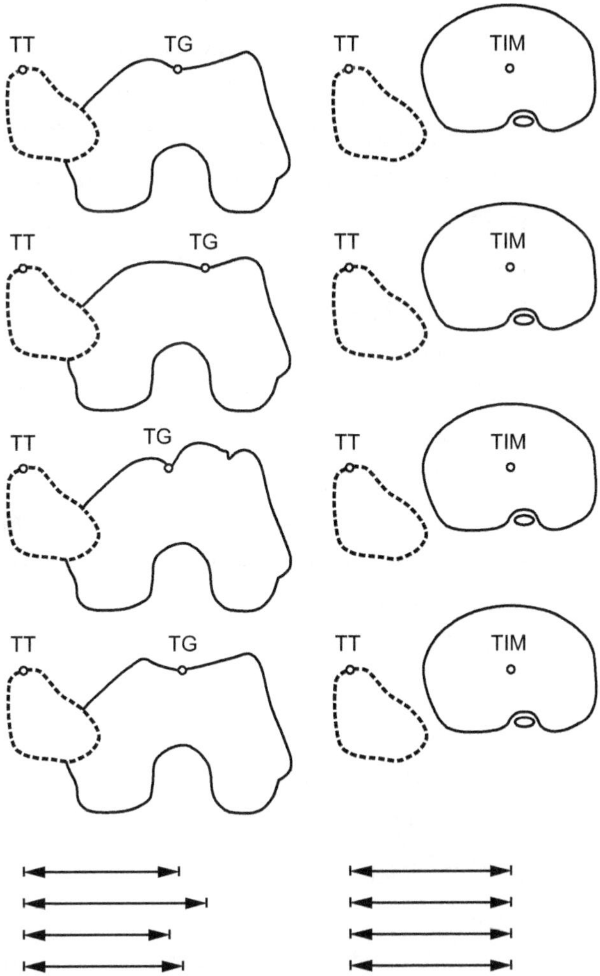

TG.................. (femoral) trochlear groove (point)
TIM .... tibial intercondylar midpoint
TT ....tibial tuberosity

Fig. 22. Anatomical (bony) positions of points reflecting the relative middle of the knee regarding the quadriceps insertion (the tibial tuberosity) if the insertion were static

With no intention to digress into TT-TG distance and its shortcomings, it has been known TT-TG distance *increases* due to *medialization* of the TG point instead of lateralization of the TT point (Paiva *et al.*, 2021, pp. 970, 972–3). Some authors have been able to demonstrate TT-TG distance *decreases* in weight-bearing conditions on upright CT imaging (Hirschmann *et al.*, 2015). However, at least for the latter, and judging from the images in their paper (Fig. 2, p. 3400), the authors have used knees *without* FTD. It also appears they did not use the 'Roman arch' cut (*see* further, p. 114) to assume the trochlear shape and define the location of TG point (Fig. 23). When femoral trochlea has a regular shape, its lowest point, the 'bottom', and hence the TG point may indeed reflect the relative middle of the intercondylar femur/the knee, which would enable the static quality of the TG point, therefore *decreasing* the TT-TG distance with quadriceps belly contraction. The problem is, however—and this is so well documented to be beyond referencing—most of recurrent patellar dislocators *have FTD.* Therefore, the surest way to circumvent this problem altogether is to have an indicator that is not influenced by FTD, such as, for example, TT-TIM distance.*

* TT-TG distance significantly depends on the femoral reference point (Tscholl *et al.*, 2016) and cannot accurately predict dynamic lateral displacement of the patella (Carlson *et al.*, 2017). Lateral patellar displacements are of main interest here, of course, because superior and medial dislocations are so exceedingly rare that only few cases have been reported (Cusco *et al.*, 2009; Miller *et al.*, 1991). To boot, TT-TG distance has different values on CT and MRI (Tan *et al.*, 2020). For more on TT-TG distance *see*, for example, an instructional review of Krishnan *et al.*, 2022.

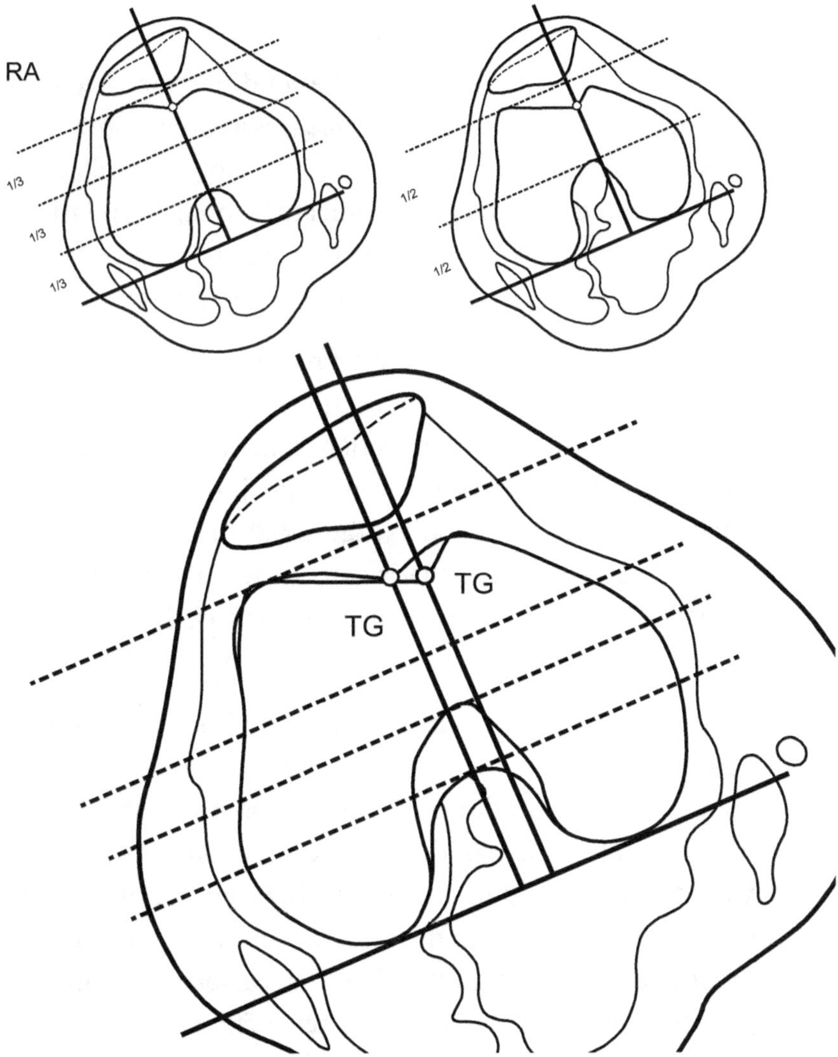

RA .... 'Roman arch'
TG.................. (femoral) trochlear groove (point)

Fig. 23. Defining the 'bottom' of the femoral trochlear groove by the TG point on different CT images

Upon defining the indicator and the condition, one needs to take care of confounders. A *confounder* is a variable influencing either an indicator or a condition. Therefore, a confounder is an unwanted intruder to the indicator–condition relationship, a third party. A total number of confounders is finite, although it might seem infinite because it is unknown.

As defined in classical mechanics, a mechanical system, a *mechanism*, is defined as such a collection of material points (particles) or bodies in which the position or motion of each particle or body of the system depends on the position and motion of all the other particles or bodies (Targ, 1988, p. 366). In biomechanics, one regards the quadriceps muscle as a mechanical system of its parts. The quadriceps muscle is, therefore, the 'quadriceps mechanism'.

One could imagine a mechanism as a set of four gears shown in Fig. 24. The movement of the first one, sets the second in motion. Then the motion of the second moves the third, and, finally, the movement of the third sets the fourth in motion. All of this happens simultaneously. In brief: if a single gear moves, **they all move**. In the mechanism, each gear is an *internal* confounder to the other. In statistical terms, this means their movements (rotations, *see* further) affect each other. This mutual confounding merely proves they are parts of the same mechanism, which is, indeed, true.

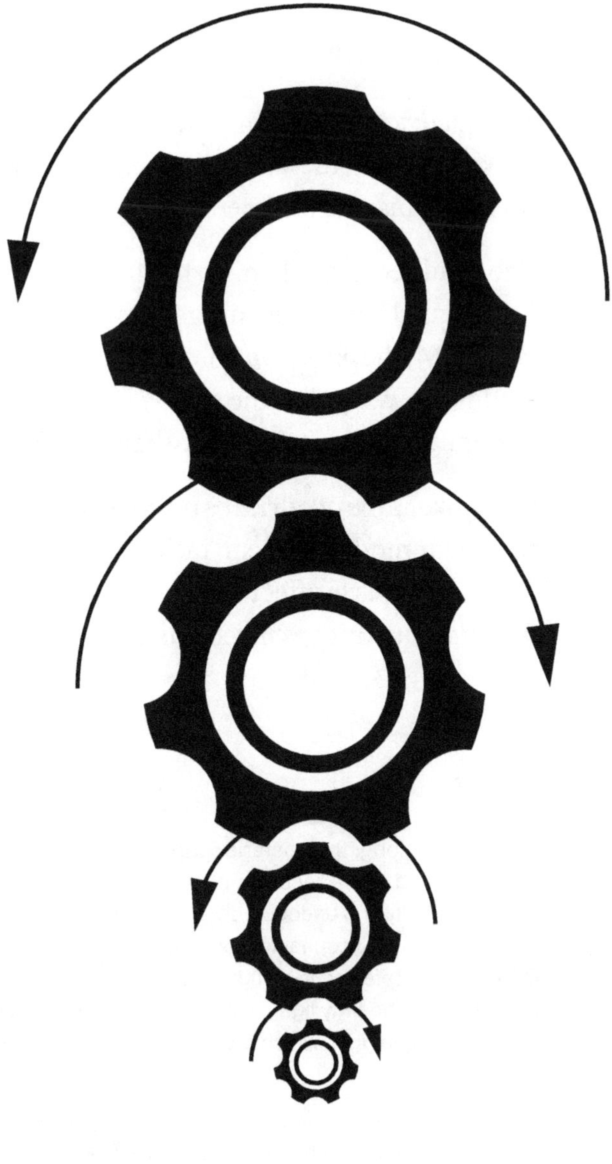

Fig. 24. Gears as a mechanism

The quadriceps mechanism is the main *extensor* of the leg in the knee, and is, therefore, frequently referred to as the 'extensor mechanism of the knee'.

The quadriceps mechanism has four parts: 1) the *origin*, 2) the *belly* ('quadriceps' meaning 'four heads' in Latin), 3) the *tendon*, and 4) the *insertion* (the tibial tuberosity). The quadriceps tendon, however, has the *superior* and *inferior* part, with the triangular bone *patella* in between (Fig. 25).*

If one likens the quadriceps mechanism to the aforementioned four-gear model, one can quickly understand that if movements of its parts affect each other, this proves they belong to the same, quadriceps mechanism, which is, indeed, true.**

* For long, the posterior part of the tendon was called the 'patellar ligament', and, more recently, as well as inacurately, the 'patellar tendon'. Microscopically, it is undoubtedly a tendon. So, macroscopically, it should be likewise because it connects the muscle with the bone (the tibia). In this small CT study, it is referred to as the 'inferior part of the quadriceps tendon'. This is not trivial: a healthy ligament needs to be elastic, whereas a healthy tendon needs to be rigid, which are, quite obviously, two diametrically opposed therapeutic goals.

** Therefore, to find a large correlation between the movements of the parts of the same mechanism is not a 'bad' result *per se* but, in fact, a proof they belong to the same mechanism.

a.......... rectus femoris muscle
b....... vastus lateralis obliquus muscle
c...... vastus medialis obliquus muscle
d............... superior part of the quadriceps tendon
e...... the patella (the kneecap)
f.................. inferior part of the quadriceps tendon
g............................... insertion (the tibial tuberosity)

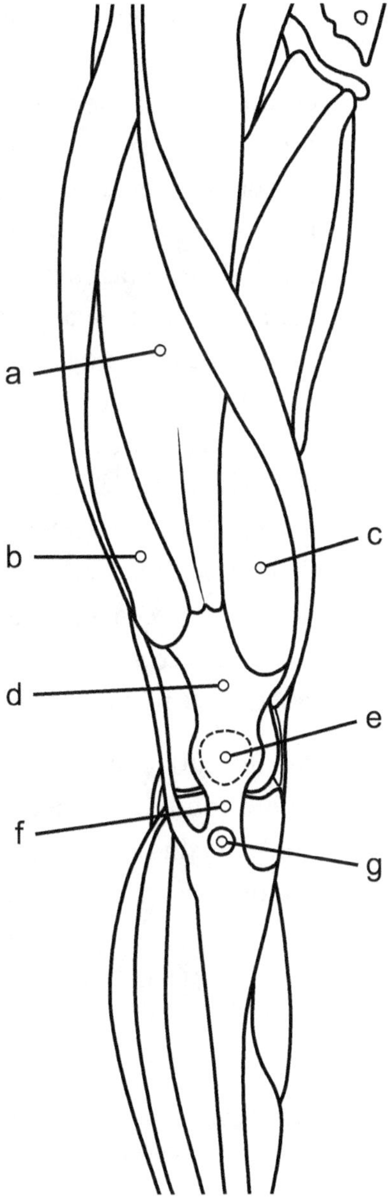

Fig. 25. Quadriceps mechanism

Patella, nonetheless, is **not** an *independent* bone. It is the largest *sesamoid* (tendon) bone* in the human body, which means it is encapsulated in the quadriceps tendon. The quadriceps muscle is the strongest muscle in the human body, and patella, quite obviously, is left to the tender mercies of its mechanism. Focusing the stability research on the patella merely because it is the leading protagonist of a dislocation would mean exaggerating its biomechanically important, yet by no means dominant role in the complex environment of knee stability. Since a muscle consists of a belly and a tendon, the patella, being a bony part of the quadriceps tendon, is hence a part of the muscle. In the quadriceps mechanism, therefore, all of its parts are not equally important. For knee stability, the *active* motion of the belly and the tendon is more important than the *passive* motion of the patella. In addition, the action of the muscle's unified vector is *maximized* at the insertion point, the tibial tuberosity (a reference point of the indicator, the TT-TIM distance).

An indicator of knee stability should reflect **the action of the whole quadriceps mechanism** by concentrating on the position of its single point, its **insertion** (the point of the maximal vector impact). Therefore, it should not be influenced, at least not to a large extent ($d < .80$ and $r < .50$) by the *separate* actions of its parts (Fig. 26).

* A sesamoid bone is found in a muscle tendon which is a fact reflected in anatomic nomenclature of certain languages. For example, a *sesamoid bone* is 'Sehnenbein' in German and 'tetivna kost' in Croatian—literally: a 'tendon bone'.

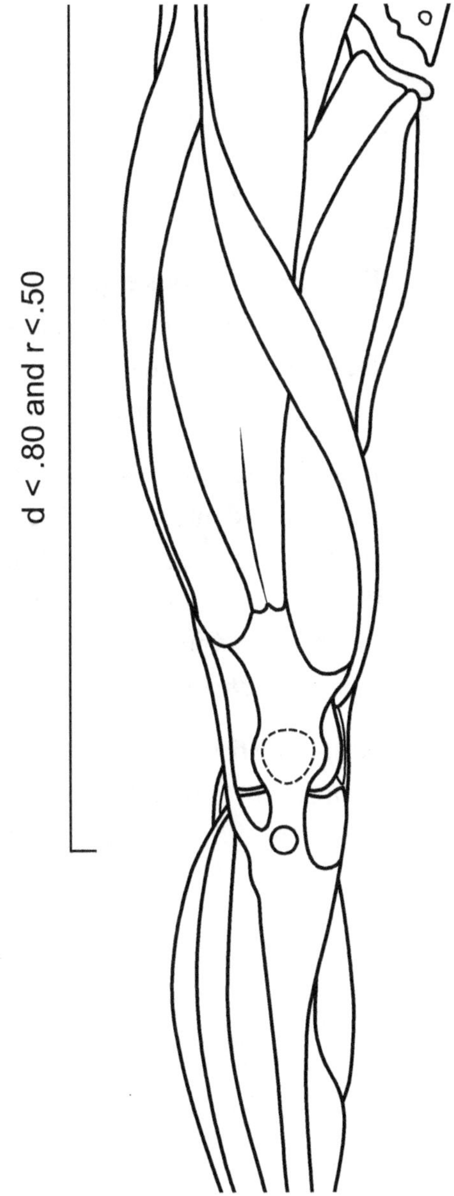

d, r...... magnitude (effect size)

Fig. 26. Expected magnitudes (effect sizes) of the relationship of the insertion (and hence the indicator) with the muscle (the belly and the tendon) and the patella

Based on previous explanations, it is now obvious there are *external* and *internal* confounders. External confounders are those *outside* the quadriceps mechanism whereas internal confounders are those *inside* the quadriceps mechanism (Fig. 27).

In logical terms, this means the confounding effects of both external and internal confounders to the indicator–condition relationship must be *excluded.* In statistical terms, this means the *differences and correlations* regarding both external and internal confounders to the indicator–condition relationship must have *theoretical* importance.

Following this line of reasoning will prove: 1) the indicator is *exclusive* to the quadriceps mechanism, and 2) the condition is *caused* by the quadriceps mechanism.

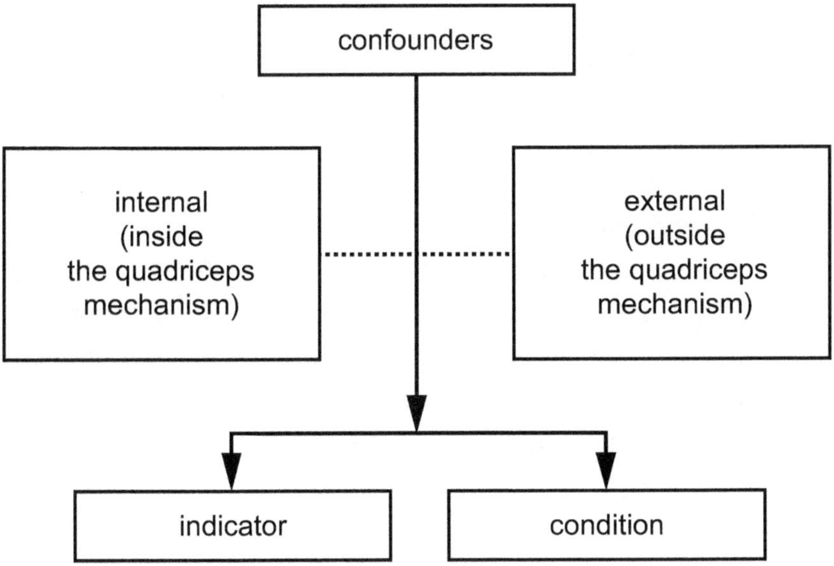

Fig. 27. Types of confounders

It is necessary to exclude a confounding effect of an *external* confounder. Its confounding effect must be excluded with regard to the indicator, but also the condition, to ensure indicator–condition relationship is exclusive.

In this small CT study, an external confounder was excluded either *directly*, by *physically* excluding an external confounder from the study, or *indirectly*, by *statistically* excluding its confounding effect on the indicator and the condition proving its theoretical importance for the indicator and the condition (Fig. 28). For example, the knees with meniscal ruptures were physically excluded from the study, as these may cause rotational disorders that might have a confounding effect to the indicator–condition relationship. On the other hand, the confounding effect of bone rotations was statistically excluded by proving its theoretical importance for the indicator and the condition.

If a single word would be necessary to describe the logical concept of dealing with external confounders, it might as well be 'sifting'.*

* The entire process of excluding the external confounders is much like a diagnosis *per exclusionem*: when every other possibility is excluded, that what is left in the end is the diagnosis, no matter how surprising it may appear. Likewise, when every theoretically important relationship is excluded, that what is left is important, and worth of interpretation and further research.

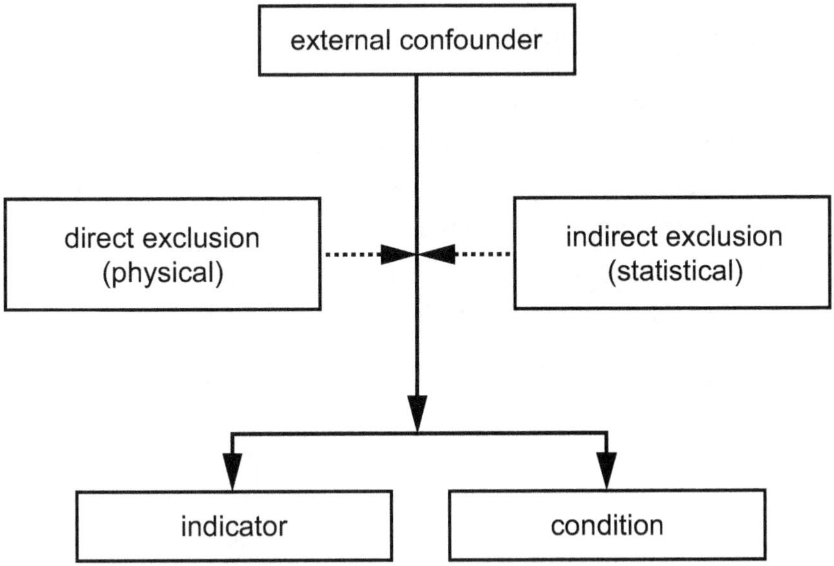

Fig. 28. Exclusion of external confounders

The *external* confounders such as:

- skin and subcutaneous tissue tumors
- femoral, tibial, and patellar fractures
- bipartite and multipartite patellae
- muscle and tendon tears
- ligament laxity and tears, and
- meniscal lesions or tears *

were *directly* excluded in both *negatives and positives* (Fig. 29).

* It is a known fact meniscal lesions are highly prevalent in both primary as well as recurrent patellar dislocators. Hence, meniscal injuries were clinically excluded from the study in both negatives and positives. For more on meniscal injuries and patellar dislocations *see*, for example, Perez *et al.*, 2024, p. 4.

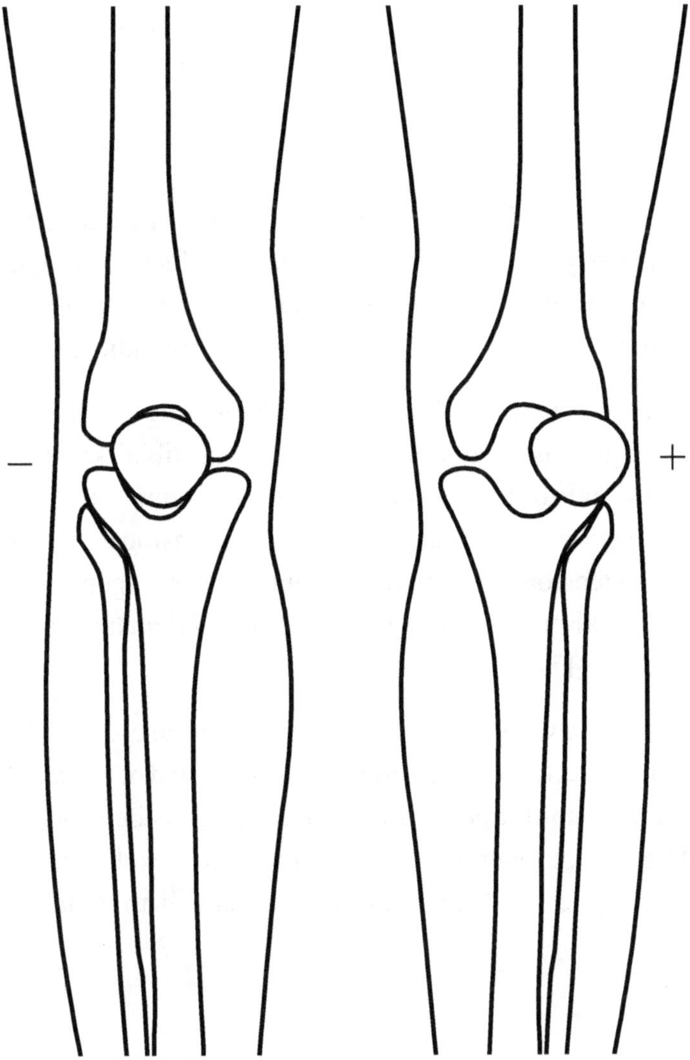

Fig. 29. Negative and positive knee

Many external confounders were *indirectly* excluded, that is to say they were *statistically* tested to exclude its confounding effect on the indicator and the condition proving its *theoretical* importance for the indicator as well as the condition.

These external confounders could be roughly divided into three groups:1) *bone rotations* (femoral/tibial/knee rotation and tibial torsion at the level of tibial tuberosity) 2) *bone deformities* (sulcus angle for FTD, extension angle for flexion-extension deformity, and joint line convergence angle for varus-valgus deformity), and 3) *general data* (age, body side and sex) (Fig. 30).

Combined with the aforementioned external confounders that were directly excluded, they make a long list of at least twenty external confounders whose influence has been addressed. The total number of external confounders excluded might be even higher due to the usage of knee pairs in the study design.

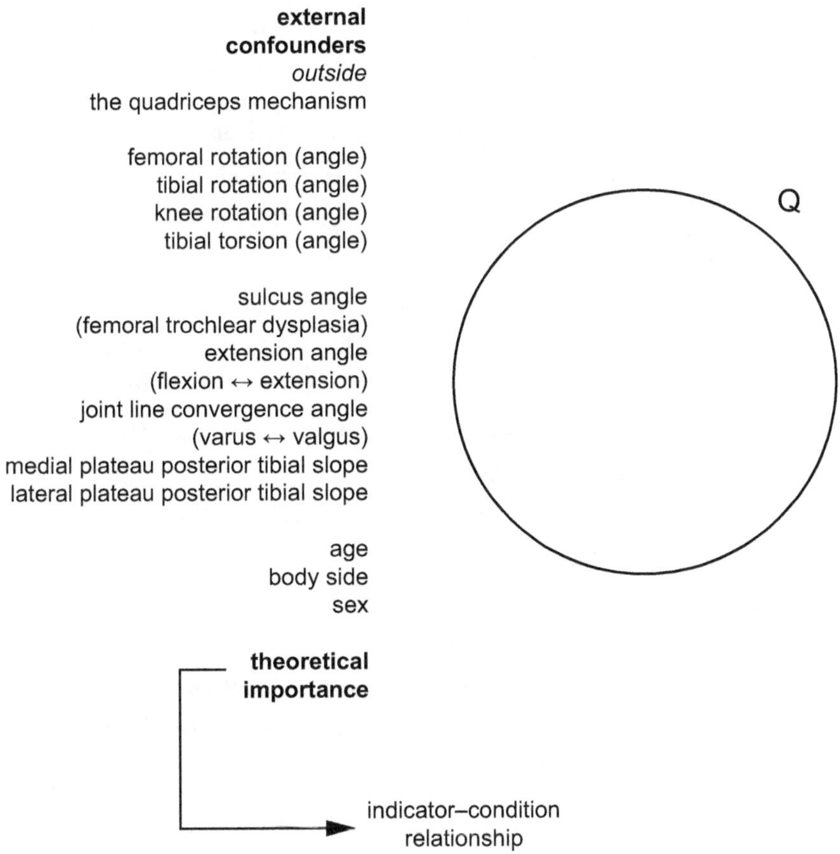

Q..... quadriceps mechanism

Fig. 30. External confounders to the indicator–condition relationship

A specific type of an external confounder was the *position of a leg during CT imaging.* On closer inspection, it comes down to bone positioning that could be either *voluntary* or *anatomical.*

Voluntary bone positioning was the position of the bone with regard to the CT table (a horizontal) (reflected by the *femoral rotation* as the angle between the posterior parts of the femur at the level of the 'Roman arch' and the horizontal, as well as the *tibial rotation* as the angle between the posterior parts of the tibia at the level of the 'headless cut' and the horizontal) (Dejour *et al.*, 1987, pp. 37–8). Voluntary bone positioning could be adjusted because it was not innate to the participant but a result of the participant's voluntary action. Due to practical reasons, however, the participants were told to keep their feet tightly together. On the other hand, *anatomical bone positioning* was the position of the bone with regard to one another (reflected by the *knee rotation* as the angle between the posterior parts of the femur and the tibia), as well as the position of the parts of the same bone with regard to one another (reflected in the *tibial torsion* as the angle between the posterior parts of the tibia at the level of the 'headless cut' and the posterior parts of the tibia at the level of the 'prominent cut') (Dejour *et al.*, 1987, pp. 37–8). Anatomical bone positioning could not be adjusted because it was innate to the participant.

The bone rotation angles are shown in Fig. 31.

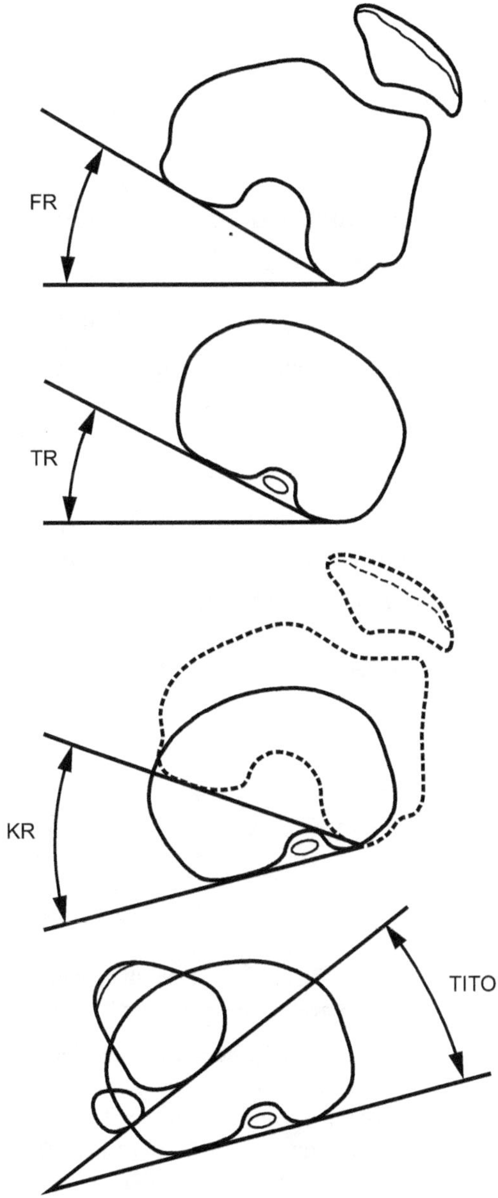

FR .... femoral rotation (angle)
KR .... knee rotation (angle)
TITO ....tibial torsion (angle) (at the level of the tibial tuberosity)
TR ....tibial rotation (angle)

Fig. 31. Bone rotation angles

To be able to define the spatial position of a bone, one needs to define *space*. Unfortunately, space is *abstract*.

Its most widely used presentation is that of three mutually vertical planes—the *frontal*, the *transverse* (axial), and the *sagittal* plane*—called the *orthogonal coordinate* ('Cartesian') *system*.**

In each plane, one theorizes a parallel coordinate, an axis, with two types of movement: *translation*, **along** the axis, and *rotation*, **around** the axis.

The orthogonal coordinate system is shown in Fig. 32.

* There is a plethora of synonyms used to denote these three planes. For this booklet, I have chosen the ones I deem most appropriate.

** Note the point where all axes intersect is called the *origin* (*o*), and is always in the *center* (the *middle*) of the orthogonal coordinate system. Therefore, it is an *absolutely static* point. The system is named after Renatus Cartesius, alias René Descartes (1596–1650), a French phylosopher and mathematician.

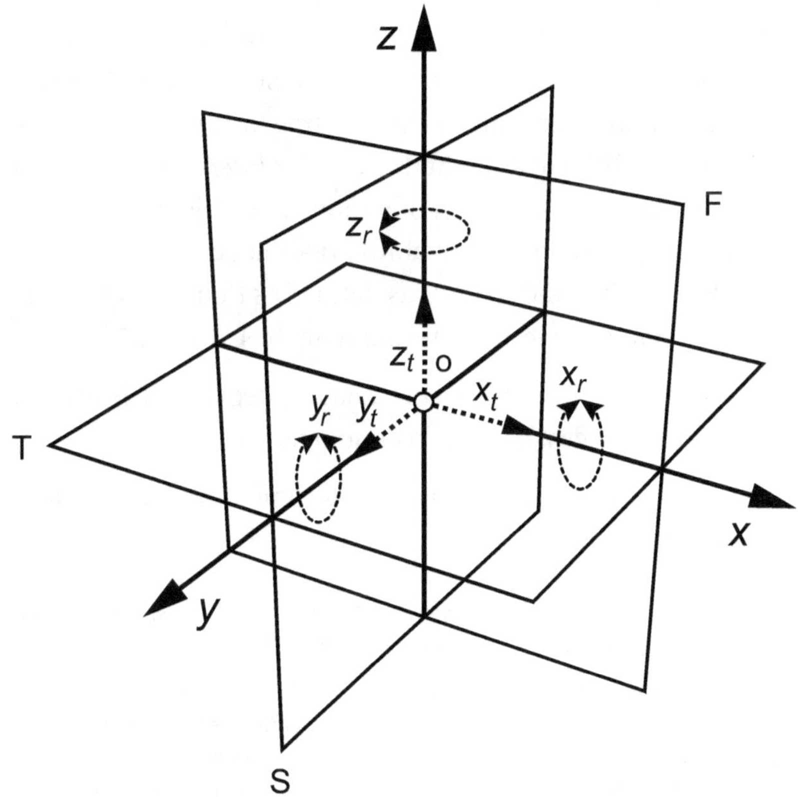

T ..... transverse (axial) plane
F .... frontal plane
S .... sagittal plane

o.................................. origin
r .... rotation
t............................ translation
x-y-z............................ axes (of the orthogonal coordinate system)

Fig. 32. Orthogonal coordinate system

In classical mechanics, the idea of an *absolutely immovable*, universal orthogonal coordinate system was introduced by Sir Isaac Newton (1643–1727) in the 17th century by use of an astronomical coordinate system with the Sun in the middle and three mutually vertical axes connecting the immovable stars (Čaušević, 2000, p. 4). It had to be *absolutely immovable* to allow relative description of a moveable object. However, in Nature, absolute immovability does not exist. To accommodate for this, the space was defined as Euclidean,* that is to say *equal* in all its parts throughout the Universe.**

Nowadays, the orthogonal coordinate system is widely used in technical sciences, but also in radiologic imaging.***

An example of triplanar view in the technical drawing of a sink is shown in Fig. 33.

* Euclid (*Εὐκλείδης, ου, ὁ*) (≈300 BC), ancient Greek mathematician, from *εὐ-κλεής*: *glorious* (Gorski and Majnarić, 2005, p. 169).

** As explained earlier, the origin is a *static* point. Any other point in the orthogonal coordinate system with its planar coordinates (*x-y-z*) is a *dynamic* point because it can change its position within the system. So, there you have a pair of points: one *static* (the origin) and one *dynamic* (the point positioned somewhere in the system). This pair of points (movable—immovable) is *vital* because to describe the motion of the point in the orthogonal coordinate system actually means to *describe its position relative to the origin*. To be able to do that, the origin itself **must be static**. Now, translate this concept to the 'wall and ball theory', where there are also two points: one *static* (the absolute/relative middle of the leg/knee) and one *dynamic* (the quadriceps mechanism insertion/the tibial tuberosity)! **This makes it very clear the former must be static for one to be able to describe the motion of the latter.** What is more, the origin of the orthogonal coordinate system may be *interchanged* with the absolute/relative middle of the leg/knee.

*** In fact, multiplanar imaging *is* the crux of radiologic imaging.

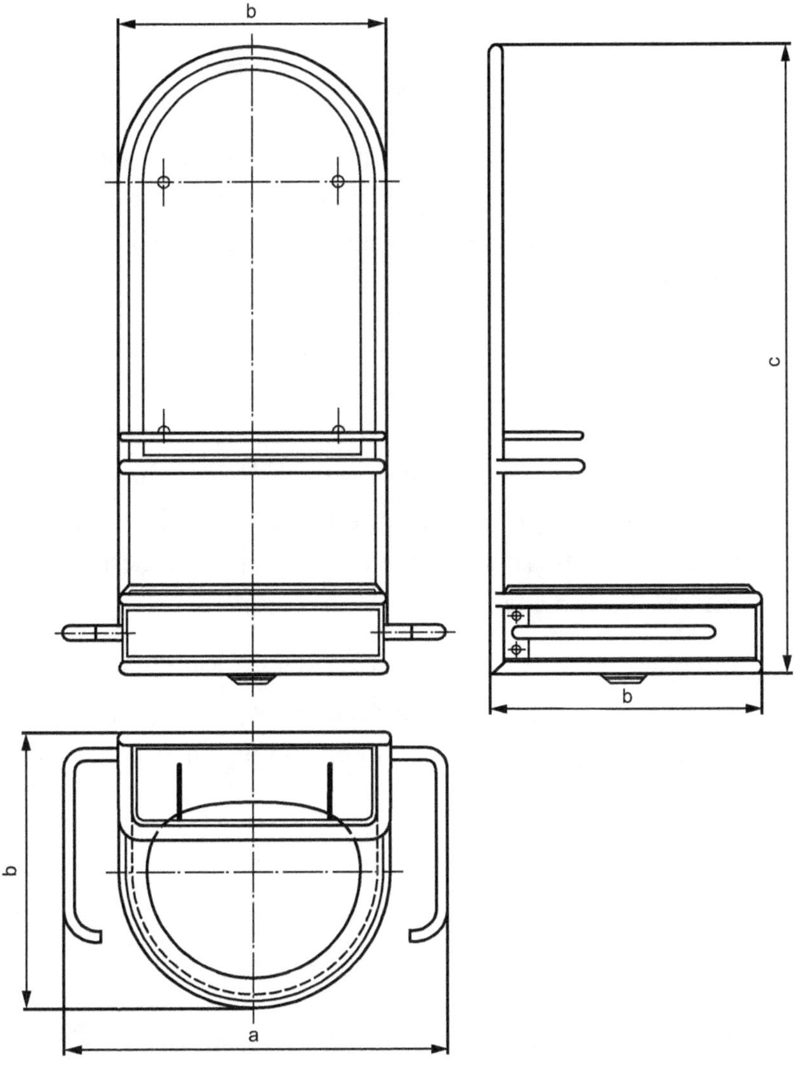

Fig. 33. Technical drawing (a sink)

In radiology, *initial* plane of imaging is the *transverse* (*axial*) *plane* whereas other imaging planes are *reconstructed* (Fig. 34).* This is why measurements are performed in the transverse (axial) plane.

The imaging is two-dimensional, although it creates a three-dimensional illusion. This is why a plane contains a *figure* rather than a body. Apart from that, it is crucial to remember a *point* in the frontal plane becomes a *vertical line* in the transverse plane! This is why one refers to *points* (thinking about the frontal plane), yet draws *vertical lines* (while projecting these points in the transverse plane).

In a plane, *translation* is reported as a *distance* in *millimeters* (mm)** whereas *rotation* is reported as an *angle* in *degrees* (°), and there is a special type of reasoning when it comes to its *direction.*

* A term CAT ('**C**omputed **A**xial **T**omography') scan comes to mind here. Transverse (axial) plane is, therefore, considered, *the* imaging plane.

** From a viewpoint of an orthopedic surgeon, only an *integer* value makes practical sense. Therefore, reporting the measurements with two or even three decimals is overkill, and brings nothing substantial to the table.

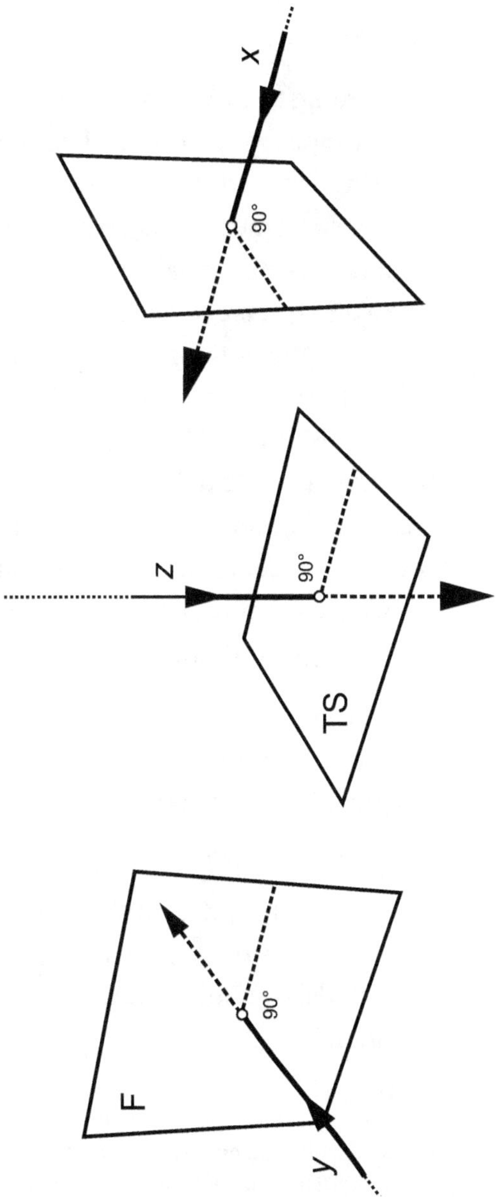

T .... transverse (axial) plane
F .... frontal plane
S ....sagittal plane
x-y-z............................ axes
(of the orthogonal
coordinate system)

Fig.34. Imaging planes

In the orthogonal coordinate system, there is a *positive* (+) and a *negative* (–) rotation of a figure in a plane.*

According to the way *direction* of rotation is regarded, there is a *left* ('clockwise' or 'French'), and *right* ('counter-clockwise' or 'English') orthogonal coordinate system. The pioneer researchers of the patellar stability field are French. In thus preferable left orthogonal coordinate system, in the frontal plane, the axes *x-y-z* are ordered in such a way that *x* is the *transverse* axis, *y* is the *anteroposterior* axis, and *z* is the *vertical* axis. Since the rotation is directed from *x* to *y*, from *y* to *z*, and from *z* to *x*, it is directed from *left to right*, hence the *left* orthogonal coordinate system. In addition, if *z*-axis were the Earth's rotational axis, and *x-y* plane the equatorial plane, then the *right* orthogonal coordinate system would be the *northern* whereas the *left* orthogonal coordinate system would be the *southern* orthogonal coordinate system (Andrejev, 1971, p. 15).

To better understand the left system, one can imagine a bolt rotating to the left, that is to say, in the *clockwise* direction (Bazjanac, 1966, p. 30) (Fig. 35).

Therefore, in the left orthogonal coordinate system, a rotation of a figure in a plane directed from left to right would be regarded as *positive* (+) whereas the rotation of a figure in a plane directed from right to left would be regarded as *negative* (–) rotation.

* One could regard the construction of different bone angles in a transverse (axial) imaging plane as an analysis of a planar geometric motion of a solid two-dimensional figure (*see*, e.g., Bazjanac, 1977, p. 151–2).

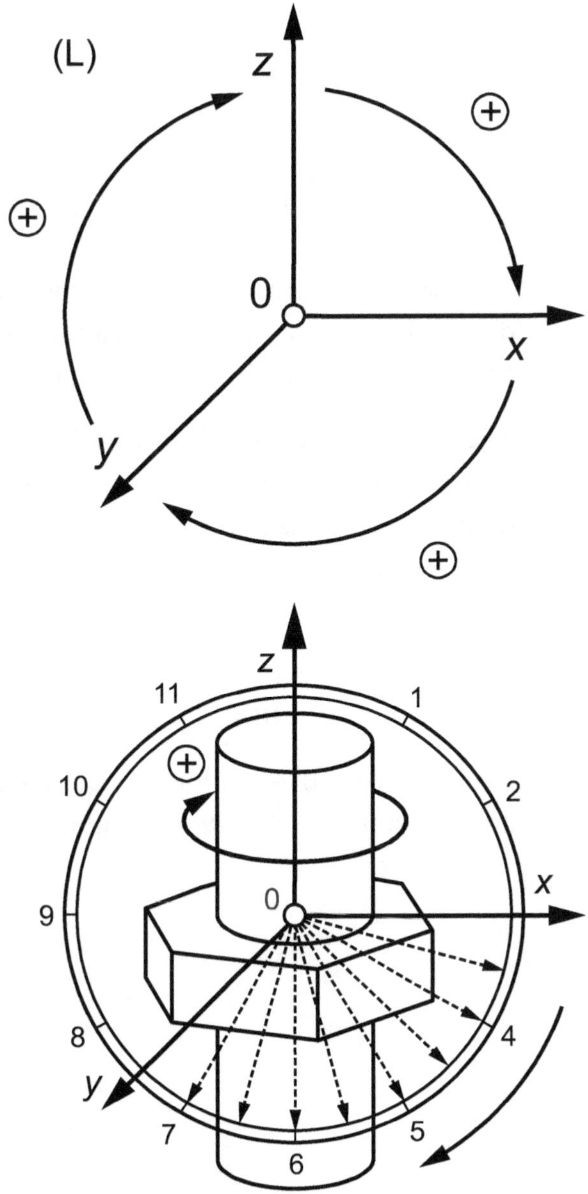

–/+ .... direction of rotation
L............................left
x-y-z.................... axes (of the orthogonal coordinate system)

Fig.35. Direction of rotation

Now, with a background in classical mechanics, it is easy to understand why *external* rotation of a bone is positive (+) whereas an *internal* rotation of a bone is negative (–) (Fig. 36).

The *knee rotation* is the difference between the femoral, and the tibial rotation angle. Given that the difference is of interest here, it is especially important to carefully note the – / + signs in order to avoid calculation error as they could lead to differing results. For example:

–15 – (–10) = –15 + 10 = **–5**, but
–15 – (+10) = –15 – 10 = **–25**.

Irrespective of the rotational direction, however, a rotation around *z*-axis, the *z-rotation*, is called a *yaw*.

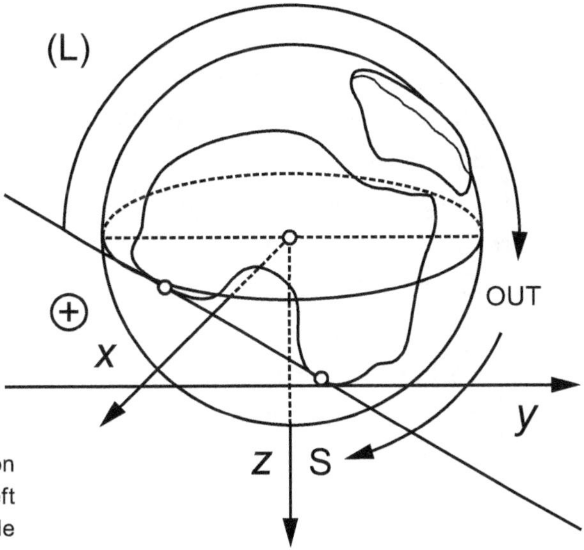

–/+ ... direction of rotation
L .... left
S .... South Pole
x-y-z .... axes
(of the orthogonal
coordinate system)

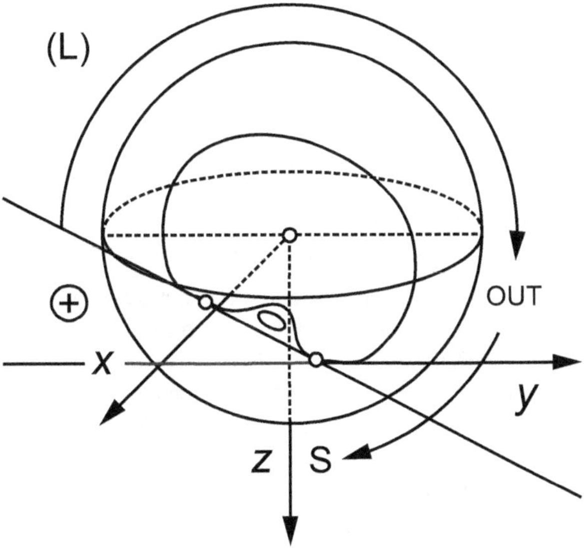

Fig. 36. Direction of bone rotation

In theory (upper part of the Fig. 37), the yaw of each bone, either with regard to the horizontal (x-axis in the transverse plane) or to one another, equals *zero*. In practice (lower part of the Fig. 37), on the other hand, a bone yaws differently with regard to the horizontal (x-axis in the transverse plane), and to each other. In fact, even a part of a bone yaws with regard to other part of the same bone (for example, tibial tuberosity with regard to the proximal part of the tibia).* All of the aforementioned bone rotation angles are, in essence, **bone yaws**.

A bone yaw is a possible external confounder of the indicator–condition relationship.** Due to practical reasons, if no large magnitude of effect to the indicator–condition relationship is present, one can conclude external confounding of a yaw is excluded.***

* In the relevant literature, the yaw is mostly referred to as 'tilt', which is a general term such as 'inclination', irrespective of a plane. With yaw, however, one is more specific as it refers to the tilt in the *transverse* plane.

** It is also a source of enormous confusion. Many studies have found an effect of various magnitudes between a bone yaw and either the indicator they studied, say TT-TG distance, or the condition. The problem begins when one needs to *contextualize* the result. Numerous yaws could be calculated as well, so much so one cannot see the forest from the trees. In this obvious conundrum, the magnitude of an effect needs to be the guide which will disentangle the coil.

*** Or is, at least, of theoretical importance.

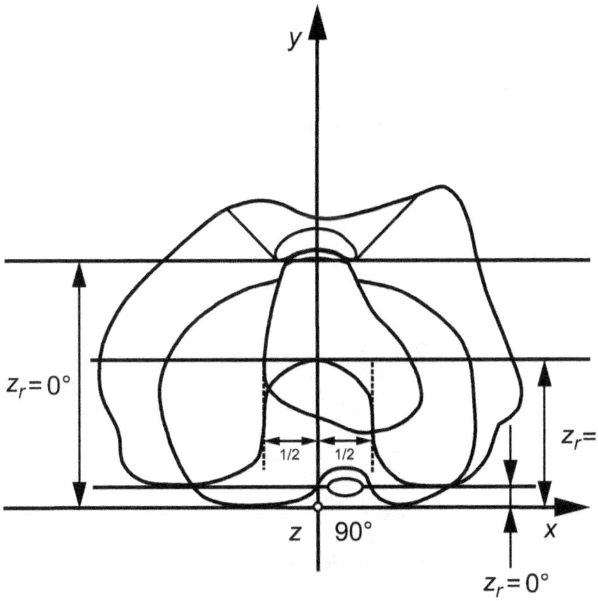

– / + ... direction of rotation
z_r...... z-rotation (yaw)
x-y-z.................. axes (of the orthogonal coordinate system)

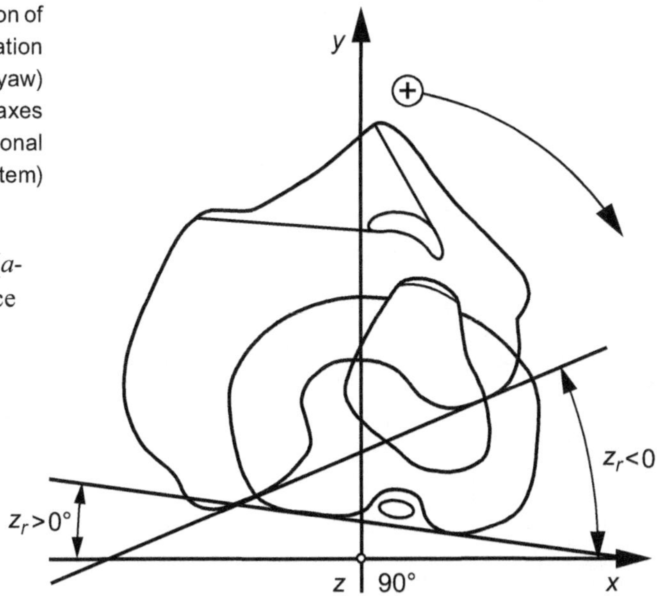

Fig. 37. Theory (*above*) and practice (*below*) of bone *z*-rotations (yaws)

The Spearman's ρ for rank correlation between the *indicator* and the *femoral rotation* was:

$$\rho = 1 - \frac{6 \times \sum d_i^2}{n \times (n^2 - 1)} = 1 - \frac{6 \times 3571}{30 \times (30^2 - 1)} = 1 - \frac{21426}{30 \times (900 - 1)}$$

$$= 1 - \frac{21426}{30 \times 899} = 1 - \frac{21426}{26970} = 1 - 0.79 = \mathbf{0.21}.$$

Given $\rho < \rho c$ (.21 < .47), the Spearman's correlation was *not statistically significant* at < .01. The magnitude was, also, 0.21.

d_i
rank difference

FR
femoral rotation
(angle)
(°)

n
sample size
(knees)

TT-TIM
tibial tuberosity
–tibial intercondylar midpoint distance
(the indicator)
(mm)

n	Relaxation		Ranks		d_i	d_i^2
	TT-TIM	*FR*	*TT-TIM*	*FR*		
1	16	−4.8	25	24.5	0.5	0.25
2	14	−5.0	14	23.0	−9	81
3	12	−13.5	5.5	14	−8.5	72.25
4	13	−10.5	8.5	17.5	−9	81
5	18	−11.4	28	15	13	169
6	15	−13.9	20.5	13	7.5	56.25
7	13	7.0	8.5	29.5	−21	441
8	14	7.0	14	29.5	−15.5	240.25
9	11	−31.0	3.5	2	1.5	2.25
10	15	−28.0	20.5	3	17.5	306.25
11	14	−14.4	14	10	4	16
12	10	−7.5	1.5	21	−19.5	380.25
13	15	−14.2	20.5	11.5	9	81
14	14	−25.8	14	5	9	81
15	11	−14.2	3.5	11.5	−8	64
16	10	−36.9	1.5	1	0.5	0.25
17	16	−3.0	25	26	−1	1
18	15	−23.3	20.5	8	12.5	156.25
19	15	−23.6	20.5	6	14.5	210.25
20	12	−22.1	5.5	9	−3.5	12.25
21	16	−5.7	25	22	3	9
22	13	−10.2	8.5	19	−10.5	110.25
23	19	4.0	29.5	28	1.5	2.25
24	14	−0.8	14	27	−13	169
25	13	−9.6	8.5	20	−11.5	132.25
26	14	−4.8	14	24.5	−10.5	110.25
27	14	−23.4	14	7	7	49
28	15	−27.8	20.5	4	16.5	272.25
29	17	−10.8	27	16	11	121
30	19	−10.5	29.5	17.5	12	144
$\Sigma d_i^2 =$						**3571**

The Spearman's ρ for rank correlation between the *indicator* and the *tibial rotation* was:

$$\rho = 1 - \frac{6 \times \sum d_i^2}{n \times (n^2 - 1)} = 1 - \frac{6 \times 3949}{30 \times (30^2 - 1)} = 1 - \frac{23694}{30 \times (900 - 1)}$$

$$= 1 - \frac{23694}{30 \times 899} = 1 - \frac{23694}{26970} = 1 - 0.88 = \mathbf{0.12.}$$

Given $\rho < \rho c$ (.12 < .47), the Spearman's correlation was *not statistically significant* at < .01. The magnitude was, also, 0.12.

d_i
rank difference

n
sample size
(knees)

TR
tibial rotation
(angle)
(°)

TT-TIM
tibial tuberosity
–tibial intercondylar midpoint distance
(the indicator)
(mm)

n	Relaxation		Ranks		d_i	d_i^2
	TT-TIM	*TR*	*TT-TIM*	*TR*		
1	16	−1.0	25	22.5	2.5	6.25
2	14	−5.4	14	17	−3	9
3	12	−11.7	5.5	8	−2.5	6.25
4	13	−10.7	8.5	9	−0.5	0.25
5	18	−9.8	28	10	18	324
6	15	−9.5	20.5	12.5	8	64
7	13	14.7	8.5	29	−20.5	420.25
8	14	17.9	14	30	−16	256
9	11	−17.6	3.5	4	−0.5	0.25
10	15	−19.3	20.5	2	18.5	342.25
11	14	4.6	14	25	−11	121
12	10	8.3	1.5	27	−25.5	650.25
13	15	−1.0	20.5	22.5	−2	4
14	14	−14.1	14	7	7	49
15	11	−1.5	3.5	21	−17.5	306.25
16	10	−21.6	1.5	1	0.5	0.25
17	16	1.6	25	24	1	1
18	15	−18.4	20.5	3	17.5	306.25
19	15	−15.0	20.5	5	15.5	240.25
20	12	−9.5	5.5	12.5	−7	49
21	16	−4.1	25	18	7	49
22	13	−14.3	8.5	6	2.5	6.25
23	19	9.7	29.5	28	1.5	2.25
24	14	5.6	14	26	−12	144
25	13	−5.7	8.5	16	−7.5	56.25
26	14	−2.2	14	20	−6	36
27	14	−3.9	14	19	−5	25
28	15	−9.7	20.5	11	9.5	90.25
29	17	−5.9	27	15	12	144
30	19	−7.7	29.5	14	15.5	240.25
$\Sigma d_i^2 =$						**3949**

The Spearman's ρ for rank correlation between the *indicator* and the *knee rotation* was:

$$\rho = 1 - \frac{6 \times \sum d_i^2}{n \times (n^2 - 1)} = 1 - \frac{6 \times 3121}{30 \times (30^2 - 1)} = 1 - \frac{18726}{30 \times (900 - 1)}$$

$$= 1 - \frac{18726}{30 \times 899} = 1 - \frac{18726}{26970} = 1 - 0.69 = \mathbf{0.31}.$$

Given $\rho < \rho c$ (.31 < .47), the Spearman's correlation was *not statistically significant* at < .01. The magnitude was, also, 0.31.

d_i
rank difference

n
sample size
(knees)

KR
knee rotation
(angle)
(°)

TT-TIM
tibial tuberosity
–tibial intercondylar midpoint distance
(the indicator)
(mm)

n	Relaxation		Ranks		d_i	d_i^2
	TT-TIM	*KR*	*TT-TIM*	*KR*		
1	16	−3.8	25	22	3	9
2	14	0.4	14	29	−15	225
3	12	−1.8	5.5	25	−19.5	380.25
4	13	0.2	8.5	28	−19.5	380.25
5	18	−1.6	28	26.5	1.5	2.25
6	15	−4.4	20.5	20	0.5	0.25
7	13	−7.7	8.5	14	−5.5	30.25
8	14	−10.9	14	11	3	9
9	11	−13.4	3.5	6	−2.5	6.25
10	15	−8.7	20.5	12	8.5	72.25
11	14	−19.0	14	2	12	144
12	10	−15.8	1.5	4	−2.5	6.25
13	15	−13.2	20.5	7	13.5	182.25
14	14	−11.7	14	10	4	16
15	11	−12.7	3.5	8	−4.5	20.25
16	10	−15.3	1.5	5	−3.5	12.25
17	16	−4.6	25	19	6	36
18	15	−4.9	20.5	17.5	3	9
19	15	−8.6	20.5	13	7.5	56.25
20	12	−12.6	5.5	9	−3.5	12.25
21	16	−1.6	25	26.5	−1.5	2.25
22	13	4.1	8.5	30	−21.5	462.25
23	19	−5.7	29.5	16	13.5	182.25
24	14	−6.4	14	15	−1	1
25	13	−3.9	8.5	21	−12.5	156.25
26	14	−2.6	14	24	−10	100
27	14	−19.5	14	1	13	169
28	15	−18.1	20.5	3	17.5	306.25
29	17	−4.9	27	17.5	9.5	90.25
30	19	−2.8	29.5	23	6.5	42.25
$\Sigma d_i^2 =$						**3121**

The Spearman's ρ for rank correlation between the *indicator* and the *tibial torsion* (at the level of the tibial tuberosity) was:

$$\rho = 1 - \frac{6 \times \sum d_i^2}{n \times (n^2 - 1)} = 1 - \frac{6 \times 4094.5}{30 \times (30^2 - 1)} = 1 - \frac{24567}{30 \times (900 - 1)}$$

$$= 1 - \frac{24567}{30 \times 899} = 1 - \frac{24567}{26970} = 1 - 0.91 = \mathbf{0.09}.$$

Given $\rho < \rho c$ (.09 < .47), the Spearman's correlation was *not statistically significant* at < .01. The magnitude was, also, 0.09.

d_i
rank difference

n
sample size
(knees)

TITO
tibial torsion at the level
of the tibial tuberosity
(angle)
(°)

TT-TIM
tibial tuberosity
–tibial intercondylar midpoint distance
(the indicator)
(mm)

n	Relaxation		Ranks		d_i	d_i^2
	TT-TIM	*TITO*	*TT-TIM*	*TITO*		
1	16	15.7	25	15	10	100
2	14	9.4	14	8	6	36
3	12	10.3	5.5	9	−3.5	12.25
4	13	11.4	8.5	11	−2.5	6.25
5	18	7.4	28	6	22	484
6	15	10.4	20.5	10	10.5	110.25
7	13	33.7	8.5	29	−20.5	420.25
8	14	37.2	14	30	−16	256
9	11	−1.0	3.5	2	1.5	2.25
10	15	−3.8	20.5	1	19.5	380.25
11	14	26.7	14	25	−11	121
12	10	29.7	1.5	28	−26.5	702.25
13	15	22.6	20.5	23	−2.5	6.25
14	14	13.2	14	12	2	4
15	11	23.9	3.5	24	−20.5	420.25
16	10	1.4	1.5	3	−1.5	2.25
17	16	21.5	25	21	4	16
18	15	5.9	20.5	5	15.5	240.25
19	15	8.2	20.5	7	13.5	182.25
20	12	14.4	5.5	13	−7.5	56.25
21	16	22.4	25	22	3	9
22	13	4.8	8.5	4	4.5	20.25
23	19	28.4	29.5	26	3.5	12.25
24	14	28.6	14	27	−13	169
25	13	17.3	8.5	18	−9.5	90.25
26	14	18.4	14	19	−5	25
27	14	15.3	14	14	0	0
28	15	16.2	20.5	16	4.5	20.25
29	17	17.1	27	17	10	100
30	19	19.4	29.5	20	9.5	90.25
$\Sigma d_i^2 =$						**4094.5**

Given T > Tc (45 > 12, n = 14), the *femoral rotation* between negatives and positives was *not statistically significant* at < .01.

The magnitude was:

d = W / S = 15 / 116 = **0.13**.

– / +
negatives and positives

†
excluded (zero) ranks

d
difference

| d |
absolute difference

FR
femoral rotation
(angle)
(°)

n
sample size
(participants)

T
smaller sum of W– and W+ ranks

W
sum of signed ranks of difference

n				FR	Ranks	Signed ranks	W−	W+
	−	+	*d*	|*d*|				
1	−5.0	−4.8	−0.2	0.2	1	−1	−1	11
2	−13.5	−10.5	−3	3	5.5	−5.5	−5.5	12
3	−13.9	−11.4	−2.5	2.5	4	−4	−4	14
4†	7.0	7.0	0	—	—	—	−5.5	13
5	−31.0	−28.0	−3	3	5.5	−5.5	−8	3
6	−7.5	−14.4	6.9	6.9	11	11	−9.5	7
7	−14.2	−25.8	11.6	11.6	12	12	−9.5	
8	−14.2	−36.9	22.7	22.7	14	14	−2	
9	−3.0	−23.3	20.3	20.3	13	13		
10	−22.1	−23.6	1.5	1.5	3	3		
11	−10.2	−5.7	−4.5	4.5	8	−8		
12	−0.8	4.0	−4.8	4.8	9.5	−9.5		
13	−9.6	−4.8	−4.8	4.8	9.5	−9.5		
14	−23.4	−27.8	4.4	4.4	7	7		
15	−10.8	−10.5	−0.3	0.3	2	−2		
116						15	**−45**	60

Given $T > Tc$ ($42 > 15$, $n = 15$), the tibial rotation between negatives and positives was *not statistically significant* at $< .01$.

The magnitude was:

$d = W / S = 36 / 120 =$ **0.30**.

– / +
negatives and positives

d
difference

| d |
absolute difference

n
sample size
(participants)

T
smaller sum of W– and W+ ranks

TR
tibial rotation
(angle)
(º)

W
sum of signed ranks of difference

n				**TR**	**Ranks**	**Signed ranks**	**W−**	**W+**
	−	+	***d***	$\lvert d \rvert$				
1	−5.4	−1.0	−4.4	4.4	9	−9	−9	1
2	−11.7	−10.7	−1.0	1.0	2	−2	−2	3
3	−9.5	−9.8	0.3	0.3	1	1	−5	7
4	14.7	17.9	−3.2	3.2	5	−5	−12	13
5	−17.6	−19.3	1.7	1.7	3	3	−8	15
6	8.3	4.6	3.7	3.7	7	7	−6	14
7	−1.0	−14.1	13.1	13.1	13	13		10
8	−1.5	−21.6	20.1	20.1	15	15		11
9	1.6	−18.4	16.8	16.8	14	14		4
10	−9.5	−15.0	5.5	5.5	10	10		
11	−14.3	−4.1	−10.2	10.2	12	−12		
12	5.6	9.7	−4.1	4.1	8	−8		
13	−5.7	−2.2	−3.5	3.5	6	−6		
14	−3.9	−9.7	5.8	5.8	11	11		
15	−5.9	−7.7	1.8	1.8	4	4		
120						36	**−42**	78

Given T > Tc (58 > 15, n = 15), the *knee rotation* between negatives and positives was *not statistically significant* at < .01.

The magnitude was:

d = W / S = –4 / 120 = **–0.03**.

– / +
negatives and positives

d
difference

| d |
absolute difference

KR
knee rotation
(angle)
(°)

n
sample size
(participants)

T
smaller sum of W– and W+ ranks

W
sum of signed ranks of difference

n				KR	Ranks	Signed ranks	W−	W+
	−	+	*d*	|*d*|				
1	0.4	−3.8	4.2	4.2	13	13	−6	13
2	−1.8	0.2	−2.0	2.0	6	−6	−9	10.5
3	−4.4	−1.6	−2.8	2.8	9	−9	−14	10.5
4	−7.7	−10.9	3.2	3.2	10.5	10.5	−5	8
5	−13.4	−8.7	−4.7	4.7	14	−14	−12	1
6	−15.8	−19.0	3.2	3.2	10.5	10.5	−2	15
7	−13.2	−11.7	−1.5	1.5	5	−5	−3	
8	−12.7	−15.3	2.6	2.6	8	8	−4	
9	−4.6	−4.9	0.3	0.3	1	1	−7	
10	−12.6	−8.6	−4.0	4.0	12	−12		
11	4.1	−1.6	5.7	5.7	15	15		
12	−6.4	−5.7	−0.7	0.7	2	−2		
13	−3.9	−2.6	−1.3	1.3	3	−3		
14	−19.5	−18.1	−1.4	1.4	4	−4		
15	−4.9	−2.8	−2.1	2.1	7	−7		
120						−4	−62	**58**

Given T > Tc (48 > 15, n = 15), the *tibial torsion* (at the level of tibial tuberosity) between negatives and positives was *not statistically significant* at < .01.

The magnitude was:

d = W / S = 24 / 120 = **0.20**.

– / +
negatives and positives

d
difference

| d |
absolute difference

n
sample size
(participants)

T
smaller sum of W– and W+ ranks

TITO
tibial torsion at the level
of the tibial tuberosity
(angle)
(°)

W
sum of signed ranks of difference

n				TITO	Ranks	Signed ranks	W−	W+
	−	+	*d*	|*d*|				
1	9.4	15.7	−6.3	6.3	11	−11	−11	7.5
2	10.3	11.4	−1.1	1.1	3.5	−3.5	−3.5	6
3	10.4	7.4	3.0	3.0	7.5	7.5	−9	7.5
4	33.7	37.2	−3.5	3.5	9	−9	−14	12
5	−1.0	−3.8	2.8	2.8	6	6	−3.5	15
6	29.7	26.7	3.0	3.0	7.5	7.5	−2	13
7	22.6	13.2	9.4	9.4	12	12	−5	10
8	23.9	1.4	22.5	22.5	15	15		1
9	21.5	5.9	15.6	15.6	13	13		
10	14.4	8.2	6.2	6.2	10	10		
11	4.8	22.4	−17.6	17.6	14	−14		
12	28.6	28.4	0.2	0.2	1	1		
13	17.3	18.4	−1.1	1.1	3.5	−3.5		
14	15.3	16.2	−0.9	0.9	2	−2		
15	17.1	19.4	−2.3	2.3	5	−5		
120						24	**−48**	72

Furthermore, the evaluation of FTD as an external confounder was based on the value of the *sulcus angle* (SA), that is to say an angle between the lines of the femoral trochlea on the transverse CT image where the 'Roman arch' was one third of the anteroposterior diameter of the bone (Fig. 38).

The values between 124° and 145° implied femoral trochlea had a *regular* shape whereas the values *greater than* 145° implied FTD (Dejour *et al.*, 1987, p. 31, Fig. 12).

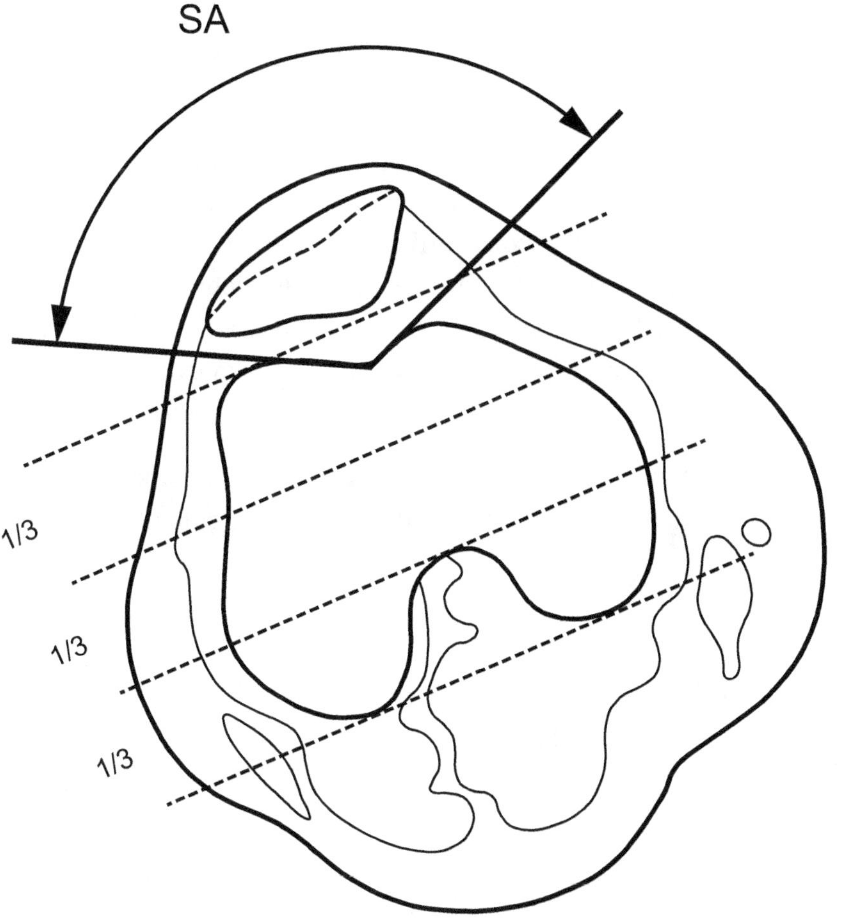

SA.....................sulcus angle

Fig. 38. Sulcus angle reflecting femoral trochlear dysplasia

The FTD was sorted according to Dejour (Tavernier and Dejour, 2001). Types A (a shallow femoral trochlea) and B (an almost flat femoral trochlea) were sorted as *mild* and types C (a dominant lateral femoral condyle) and D (a trochlear 'cliff') as *strong* FTD (Fig. 39).

Given that the original cut-off between types A and B was not provided, in this small CT study they were calculated as:

180° – 145° = 17.5°.
145° + 17.5° = 162.5°.

Therefore:

Type A = 145–162.5°.
Type B = 162.5–180°.

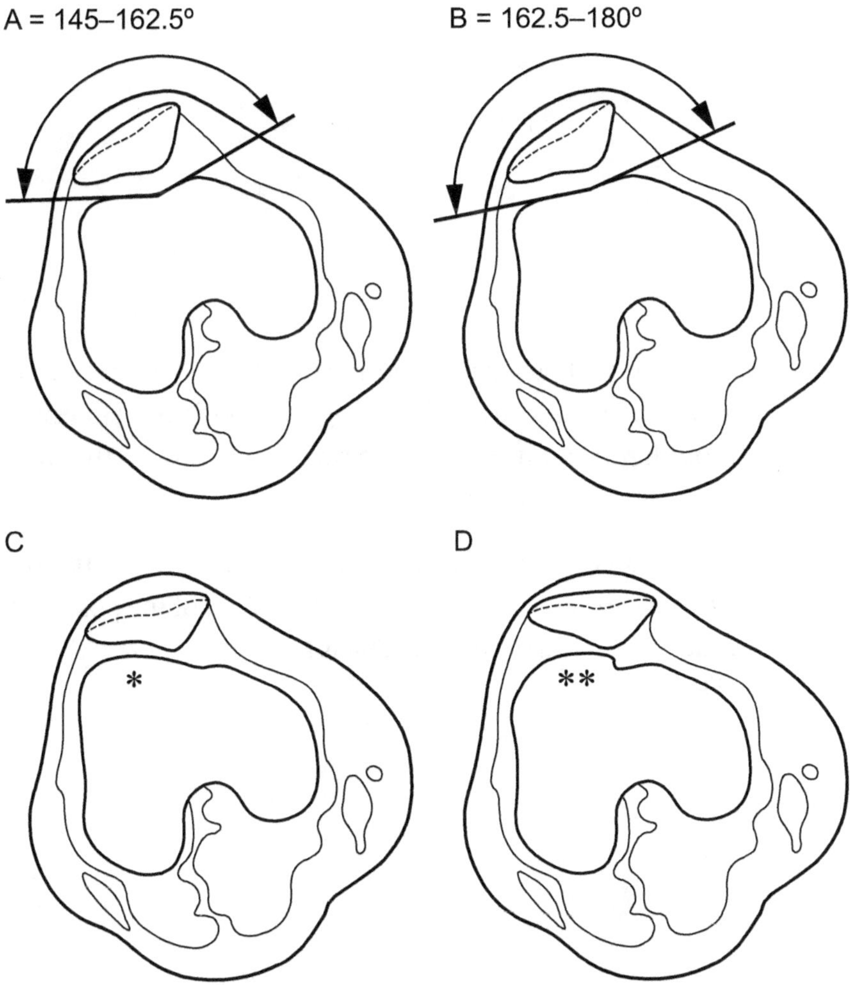

A, B, C, D ......Dejour types of femoral trochlear dysplasia
* .... dominant lateral femoral condyle
** .... trochlear cliff

Fig. 39. Dejour types of femoral trochlear dysplasia

Nowadays, we know FTD is *absent* in most (95%) of the negatives and *present* in most (70–90%) of the positives. However, although present in most of the positives, most of the time (around 80%) its has a *mild* form.

In this small CT study, as shown in table on the right, **none** of the negatives had FTD whereas **47% (7/15)** of the positives did have it, yet in a **mild** form, that is to say types A (86%; 6/7) and B (14%; 1/7).*

SA
sulcus angle
(°)

* The prevalence of nearly 50% of FTD in the sample and not 70–90% is probably due to n = 15. In larger samples one could expect this percentage to rise.

Inidividual	SA	
	–	+
1	132.6	135.3
2	138.5	130.7
3	139.4	157.1
4	142.8	172.8
5	137.6	123.6
6	131.1	125.9
7	139.2	151.7
8	143.9	155.0
9	94.9	137.8
10	128.0	137.9
11	138.2	155.9
12	136.0	146.5
13	139.8	149.6
14	140.4	141.0
15	131.2	127.3

The Spearman's ρ for rank correlation between the *indicator* and *sulcus angle* was:

$$\rho = 1 - \frac{6 \times \sum d_i^2}{n \times (n^2 - 1)} = 1 - \frac{6 \times 4608.5}{30 \times (30^2 - 1)} = 1 - \frac{27651}{30 \times (900 - 1)}$$

$$= 1 - \frac{27651}{30 \times 899} = 1 - \frac{27651}{26970} = 1 - 1.03 = \mathbf{-0.03}.$$

Given $\rho < \rho c$ (.03 < .47), the Spearman's correlation was *not statistically significant* at < .01. The magnitude was, also, – 0.03.

d_i
rank difference

n
sample size
(knees)

SA
sulcus
angle
(°)

TT–TIM
tibial tuberosity
–tibial intercondylar midpoint distance
(indicator)
(mm)

n	Relaxation		Ranks		d_i	d_i^2
	TT-TIM	*SA*	*TT-TIM*	*SA*		
1	16	135.3	25	10	15	225
2	14	132.6	14	9	5	25
3	12	138.5	5.5	16	– 10.5	110.25
4	13	130.7	8.5	6	2.5	6.25
5	18	157.1	28	29	– 1	1
6	15	139.4	20.5	18	2.5	6.25
7	13	142.8	8.5	22	– 13.5	182.25
8	14	172.8	14	30	– 16	256
9	11	137.6	3.5	12	–8.5	72.25
10	15	123.6	20.5	2	18.5	342.25
11	14	125.9	14	3	11	121
12	10	131.1	1.5	7	–5.5	30.25
13	15	139.2	20.5	17	3.5	12.25
14	14	151.7	14	26	– 12	144
15	11	143.9	3.5	23	– 19.5	380.25
16	10	155.0	1.5	27	–25.5	650.25
17	16	94.9	25	1	24	576
18	15	137.8	20.5	13	7.5	56.25
19	15	137.9	20.5	14	6.5	42.25
20	12	128.0	5.5	5	0.5	0.25
21	16	155.9	25	28	–3	9
22	13	138.2	8.5	15	–6.5	42.25
23	19	146.5	29.5	24	5.5	30.25
24	14	136.0	14	11	3	9
25	13	139.8	8.5	19	– 10.5	110.25
26	14	149.6	14	25	– 11	121
27	14	140.4	14	20	–6	36
28	15	141.0	20.5	21	–0.5	0.25
29	17	131.2	27	8	19	361
30	19	127.3	29.5	4	25.5	650.25
$\Sigma d_i^2 =$						**4608.5**

Given T > Tc (23 > 15, n = 15), the *sulcus angle* between negatives and positives was *not statistically significant* at < .01.

The magnitude was:

d = W / S = – 74 / 120 = **– 0.62**.

– / +
negatives and positives

d
difference

| d |
absolute difference

n
sample size
(participants)

SA
sulcus
angle
(°)

T
smaller sum of W– and W+ ranks

W
sum of signed ranks of difference

n				**SA**	**Ranks**	**Signed ranks**	**W–**	**W+**
	–	+	***d***	**|*d*|**				
1	132.6	135.3	–2.7	2.7	2	–2	–2	5
2	138.5	130.7	7.8	7.8	5	5	–12.5	11
3	139.4	157.1	–17.7	17.7	12.5	–12.5	–14	4
4	142.8	172.8	–30	30	14	–14	–10	
5	137.6	123.6	14	14	11	11	–9	
6	131.1	125.9	5.2	5.2	4	4	–15	
7	139.2	151.7	–12.5	12.5	10	–10	–7	
8	143.9	155	–11.1	11.1	9	–9	–12.5	
9	94.9	137.8	–42.9	42.9	15	–15	–8	
10	128	137.9	–9.9	9.9	7	–7	–6	
11	138.2	155.9	–17.7	17.7	12.5	–12.5	–1	
12	136	146.5	–10.5	10.5	8	–8		
13	139.8	149.6	–9.8	9.8	6	–6		
14	140.4	141	–0.6	0.6	1	–1		
15	131.2	127.3	3.9	3.9	3	3		
120						–74	–97	**23**

Scanning the *region of interest* (ROI) in different knee positions, however, largely differs among studies with regard to the flexion angles, which should be considered in comparing their result (Fig. 40a). For example, the original French authors used XR imaging in 30° of flexion (Goutallier *et al.*, 1978, p. 425, Fig. 2). In this small CT study, however, a participant was *supine*, scanned in extension first, with quadriceps muscles relaxed, and then during the *maximum voluntary isometric contraction* (MVIC) of the quadriceps muscles (Fig. 40b, 40c).*

It should be emphasized here, since patellar stability may be regarded as a *postural* disorder, one would benefit the most if the scanning could be performed using a magnetic resonance (MR) scanner in an *upright* position, followed by the measurement of the indicator. In the standing position, the tightness of the quadriceps muscle is somewhere between the basic muscular tonus (as in supine relaxation), and MVIC. The main goal of conservative therapy, however, would be to strengthen the postural ability of the quadriceps muscle, hence its *involuntary* (postural) isometric contraction.

* In this small CT study, therefore, the flexion scanning was not performed, though adults have a slight flexion contracture at the knee joint (Greene *et al.*, 1994, p.115). It would be beneficial to test the indicator at different angles of flexion. For example, we know TT-TG distance depends on knee flexion (Camathias *et al.*, 2016), increasing with extension (Biedert, 2004, p. 97). Given that CT and MRI values of TT-TIM distance agree (Nizić *et al.*, 2025), unlike TT-PCL, TT-RA and TT-TG distances (Irarrázaval *et al.*, 2024) although the angles of flexion are different during CT and MRI scanning, it may be plausible to hypothesize the indicator cannot be largely confounded, and might be rather stable in different degrees of flexion. It has been shown different angles of knee flexion are the very reason why CT and MRI values of TT-TG distance are not equal (Bae *et al.*, 2023).

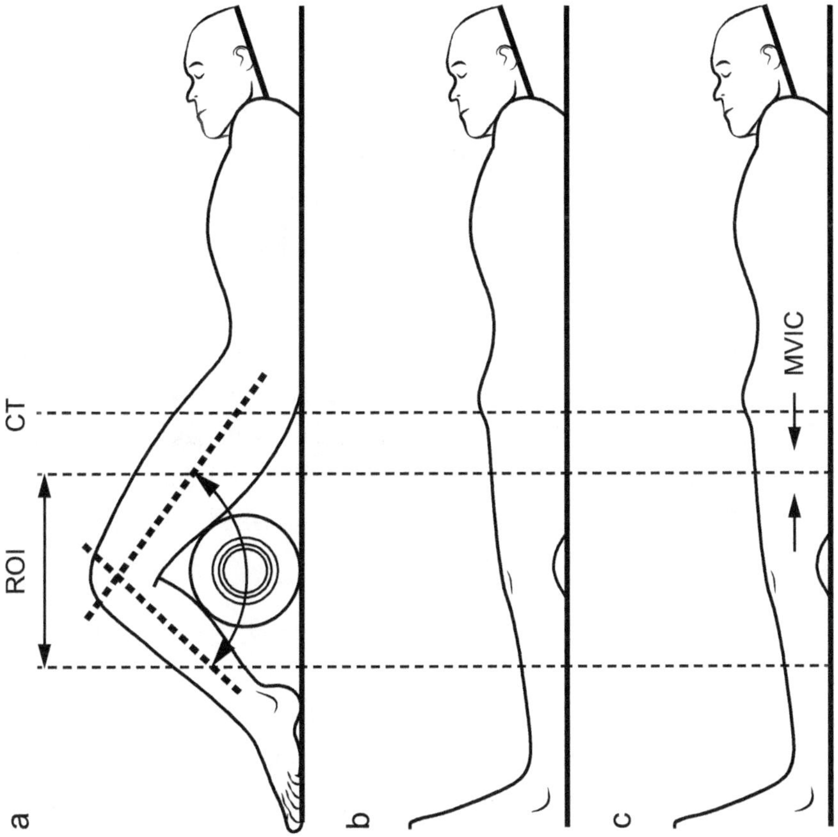

Fig. 40. Scanning positions in flexion **(a)** and extension with relaxation **(b)** or maximum voluntary isometric contraction of the quadriceps muscle **(c)**

CT.....computed tomography (scanner)
ROI..........region of interest
MVIC ....maximum voluntary isometric contraction (of the quadriceps muscle)

In this small CT study, the participants were scanned in the *supine* position, with legs in *full extension*. Hence, there was not much one could do to exclude the angle of knee flexion as a possible external confounder.

Nevertheless, the *extension angle* (EA) was measured as the angle between the cortical line of the femur and the cortical line of the tibia on reconstructed sagittal CT images with quadriceps muscles in relaxation (Paley, 2002, p. 161, Fig. 6–10). The EA was measured on a CT image exhibiting the full diameter of the femur and the tibia.

If the lines were *collinear*, the EA was *zero*. The EA closing to the right was notated as *positive* (+) because its direction of rotation was *clockwise* ('French') whereas the EA closing to the left was notated as *negative* (–) because its direction of rotation was *counter-clockwise* ('English') (*see* p. 96) (Fig. 41).*

* Whether or not there was a *hyperextension* or *fixed flexion deformity* of a knee was not the focus of this small CT study. The main intention was to test the magnitude of the relationship between the extension angle and the indicator–condition relationship.

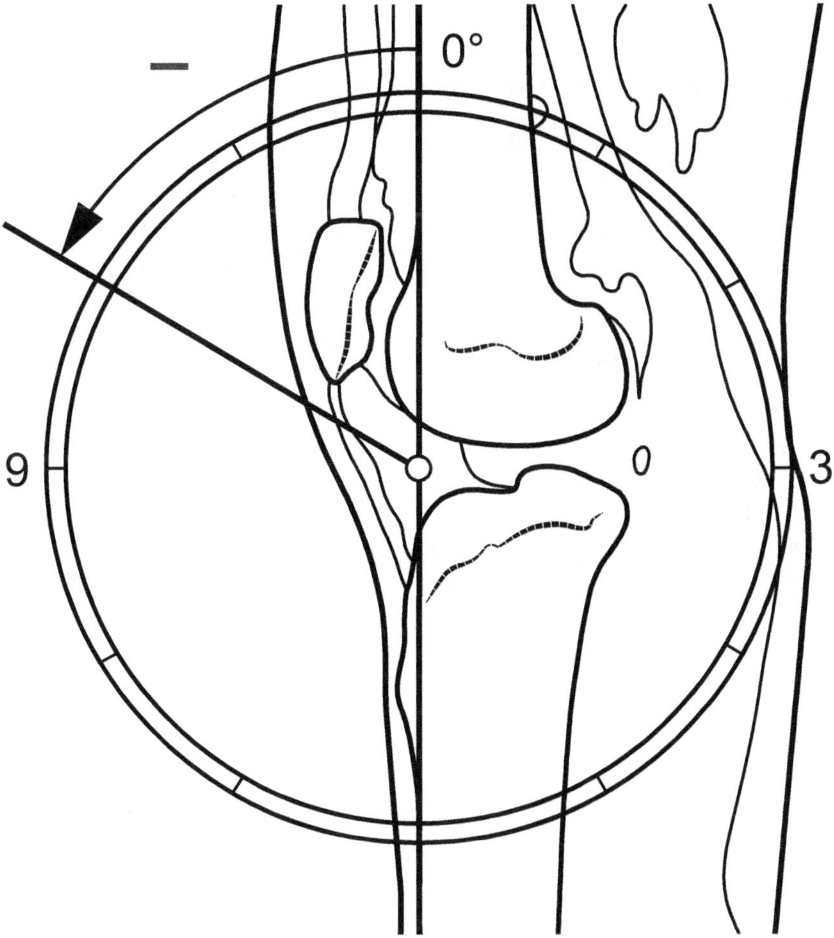

–/+ ....direction of rotation

Fig. 41. Extension angle in the sagittal plane (the direction of rotation)

The Spearman's ρ for rank correlation between the *indicator* and the *extension angle* was:

$$\rho = 1 - \frac{6 \times \sum d_i^2}{n \times (n^2 - 1)} = 1 - \frac{6 \times 5987}{30 \times (30^2 - 1)} = 1 - \frac{35922}{30 \times (900 - 1)}$$

$$= 1 - \frac{35922}{30 \times 899} = 1 - \frac{35922}{26970} = 1 - 1.33 = \mathbf{-\,0.33}.$$

Given $\rho < \rho c$ (.33 < .47), the Spearman's correlation was *not statistically significant* at < .01. The magnitude was, also, – 0.33.

d_i
rank difference

EA
extension
angle
(°)

n
sample size
(knees)

TT-TIM
tibial tuberosity
–tibial intercondylar midpoint distance
(the indicator)
(mm)

n	Relaxation		Ranks		d_i	d_i^2
	TT-TIM	*EA*	*TT-TIM*	*EA*		
1	16	−4.7	25	1.5	23.5	552.25
2	14	−3.1	14	5	9	81
3	12	−0.6	5.5	7	−1.5	2.25
4	13	−0.2	8.5	9	−0.5	0.25
5	18	−0.3	28	8	20	400
6	15	2.7	20.5	26	−5.5	30.25
7	13	2.5	8.5	24	−15.5	240.25
8	14	3.1	14	27	−13	169
9	11	2.5	3.5	24	−20.5	420.25
10	15	4.5	20.5	28	−7.5	56.25
11	14	0	14	12.5	1.5	2.25
12	10	0	1.5	12.5	−11	121
13	15	0.6	20.5	17	3.5	12.25
14	14	0.5	14	16	−2	4
15	11	1.6	3.5	21	−17.5	306.25
16	10	2.5	1.5	24	−22.5	506.25
17	16	−3.9	25	4	21	441
18	15	−1.5	20.5	6	14.5	210.25
19	15	0	20.5	12.5	8	64
20	12	1.4	5.5	19.5	−14	196
21	16	13.4	25	30	−5	25
22	13	13.2	8.5	29	−20.5	420.25
23	19	1.4	29.5	19.5	10	100
24	14	1.3	14	18	−4	16
25	13	1.7	8.5	22	−13.5	182.25
26	14	0	14	12.5	1.5	2.25
27	14	0	14	12.5	1.5	2.25
28	15	0	20.5	12.5	8	64
29	17	−4.4	27	3	24	576
30	19	−4.7	29.5	1.5	28	784
$\Sigma d_i^2 =$						**5987**

Given $T > T_c$ (45.5 > 9, n = 13), the *extension angle* between negatives and positives was *not statistically significant* at < .01.

The magnitude was:

d = W / S = 0 / 100 = **0**.

–/+
negatives and positives

†
excluded (zero) ranks

d
difference

| d |
absolute difference

EA
extension
angle
(°)

n
sample size
(participants)

T
smaller sum of W– and W+ ranks

W
sum of signed ranks of difference

n				**EA**	**Ranks**	**Signed ranks**	**W−**	**W+**
	−	+	***d***	|***d***|				
1	−3.1	−4.7	1.6	1.6	9	9	−5	9
2	−0.6	−0.2	−0.4	0.4	5	−5	−6	13
3	2.7	−0.3	3	3	13	13	−11	1.5
4	2.5	3.1	−0.6	0.6	6	−6	−7	8
5	2.5	4.5	−2	2	11	−11	−12	10
6†	0	0	0	0	—	—	−3	4
7	0.6	0.5	0.1	0.1	1.5	1.5	−1.5	
8	1.6	2.5	−0.9	0.9	7	−7		
9	−3.9	−1.5	−2.4	2.4	12	−12		
10	1.4	0	1.4	1.4	8	8		
11	13.2	13.4	−0.2	0.2	3	−3		
12	1.3	1.4	−0.1	0.1	1.5	−1.5		
13	1.7	0	1.7	1.7	10	10		
14†	0	0	0	0	—	—		
15	−4.4	−4.7	0.3	0.3	4	4		
100						0	−45.5	**45.5**

Another possible external confounder to the indicator–condition relationship with regard to the bone rotations would be a *varus–valgus deformity.*

In this small CT study, to evaluate that confounding effect, an angle formed between joint orientation lines of opposite sides of the knee in the frontal plane on reconstructed CT images, the *joint line convergence angle* (JLCA), was measured as shown in Fig. 42. (Paley, 2002, p. 8). On closer inspection, it is a *y*-rotation. The angle is simple to measure, yet a source of at least three informations: *cartilage height*, *capsular laxity*, and *varus–valgus influence* (Paley, 2002, pp. 25, 465).

It is worth highlighting, however, the values of JLCA in this small CT study reflect a *non-weightbearing, supine position.**

* It is widely accepted the normative values range between 0° and 2° medial whereas values above 2° represent a source of mechanical axis deviation (Paley, 2002, pp. 25–6, 455). Nevertheless, the values were compared as measured, and no dichotomization with regard to the varus–valgus deformity was performed. This is because a cut-off is *arbitrary*, hence it might be prudent to use raw measurements.

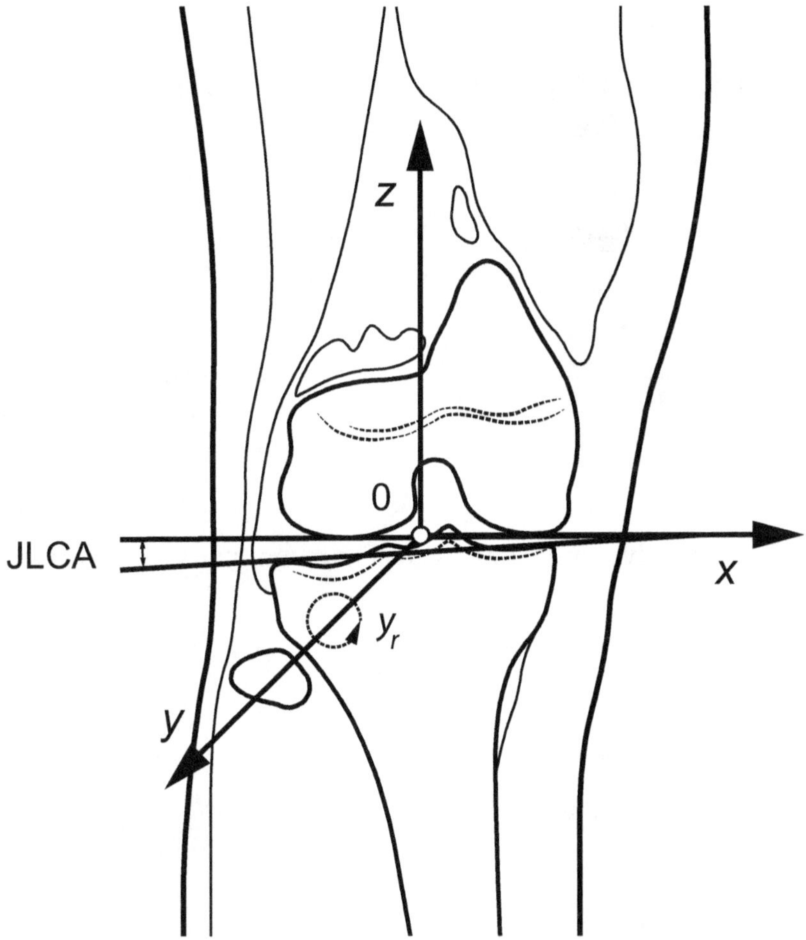

JLCA........................ joint line convergence angle (°)
x-y-z....axes (of the orthogonal coordinate system)
y_r............................ *y*-rotation

Fig. 42. Joint line convergence angle in the frontal plane

The Spearman's ρ for rank correlation between the *indicator* and the *joint line convergence angle* was:

$$\rho = 1 - \frac{6 \times \sum d_i^2}{n \times (n^2 - 1)} = 1 - \frac{6 \times 3782}{30 \times (30^2 - 1)} = 1 - \frac{22692}{30 \times (900 - 1)}$$

$$= 1 - \frac{22692}{30 \times 899} = 1 - \frac{22692}{26970} = 1 - 0.84 = \mathbf{0.16}.$$

Given $\rho < \rho c$ (.16 < .47), the Spearman's correlation was not statistically significant at < .01. The magnitude was, also, 0.16.

d_i
rank difference

JLCA
joint line convergence angle
(°)

n
sample size
(knees)

TT-TIM
tibial tuberosity
–tibial intercondylar midpoint distance
(the indicator)
(mm)

n	Relaxation		Ranks		d_i	d_i^2
	TT-TIM	*JLCA*	*TT-TIM*	*JLCA*		
1	16	−2.9	25	3.5	21.5	462.25
2	14	−1.5	14	10	4	16
3	12	−0.8	5.5	17	−11.5	132.25
4	13	−1.2	8.5	12	−3.5	12.25
5	18	−1.6	28	9	19	361
6	15	0.8	20.5	25	−4.5	20.25
7	13	1.2	8.5	27.5	−19	361
8	14	2.2	14	30	−16	256
9	11	−2.8	3.5	5	−1.5	2.25
10	15	0	20.5	22.5	−2	4
11	14	−1.0	14	14.5	−0.5	0.25
12	10	−0.1	1.5	21	−19.5	380.25
13	15	0	20.5	22.5	−2	4
14	14	−0.6	14	18	−4	16
15	11	−1.4	3.5	11	−7.5	56.25
16	10	−2.9	1.5	3.5	−2	4
17	16	−0.5	25	19	6	36
18	15	−2.1	20.5	7	13.5	182.25
19	15	−1.1	20.5	13	7.5	56.25
20	12	−1.0	5.5	14.5	−9	81
21	16	−3.0	25	2	23	529
22	13	−0.9	8.5	16	−7.5	56.25
23	19	1.5	29.5	29	0.5	0.25
24	14	1.2	14	27.5	−13.5	182.25
25	13	−1.8	8.5	8	0.5	0.25
26	14	0.2	14	24	−10	100
27	14	−3.5	14	1	13	169
28	15	−2.4	20.5	6	14.5	210.25
29	17	1.0	27	26	1	1
30	19	−0.4	29.5	20	9.5	90.25
$\Sigma d_i^2 =$						**3782**

Given T > Tc (42 > 15, n = 15), the *joint line convergence angle* between negatives and positives was *not statistically significant* at < .01.

The magnitude was:

d = W / S = 36 / 120 = **0.30**.

– / +
negatives and positives

d
difference

| d |
absolute difference

JLCA
joint line convergence angle
(°)

n
sample size (participants)

T
smaller sum of W– and W+ ranks

W
sum of signed ranks of difference

n				JLCA	Ranks	Signed ranks	W−	W+
	−	+	*d*	|*d*|				
1	−1.5	−2.9	1.4	1.4	8.5	8.5	−6	8.5
2	−0.8	−1.2	0.4	0.4	3	3	−15	3
3	0.8	−1.6	2.4	2.4	14	14	−2	14
4	1.2	2.2	−1.0	1.0	6	−6	−12	5
5	−2.8	0	−2.8	2.8	15	−15	−7	4
6	−0.1	−1.0	0.9	0.9	5	5		10
7	0	−0.6	0.6	0.6	4	4		11
8	−1.4	−2.9	1.5	1.5	10	10		1
9	−0.5	−2.1	1.6	1.6	11	11		13
10	−1.0	−1.1	0.1	0.1	1	1		8.5
11	−0.9	−3.0	2.1	2.1	13	13		
12	1.2	1.5	−0.3	0.3	2	−2		
13	−1.8	0.2	−2.0	2.0	12	−12		
14	−3.5	−2.4	−1.1	1.1	7	−7		
15	1.0	−0.4	1.4	1.4	8.5	8.5		
120						36	**−42**	78

Another possible external confounder to the indicator–condition relationship may be the *posterior tibial slope* (PTS).

In this small CT study, to evaluate that confounding effect, *medial plateau PTS* (MPTS) and *lateral plateau PTS* (LPTS) have been measured according to the method described by Hudek *et al.* in 2009, originally devised for MRI.

On the CT cut depicting *eminentia intercondylaris, posterior cruciate ligament* (PCL) attachment and concave anterior and posterior tibial cortex was defined. Then, two circles in the tibial head, the *cranial* and the *caudal* were drawn in such a way that the center of the caudal circle was on the rim of the cranial circle, both circles touching the cortex on each side. The line connecting the centers of the circles was the *tibial longitudinal axis* (TLA) which was copied and pasted on all images of the series. The PTS angle was the angle between the vertical to the TLA and the medial or the lateral plateau tangent.*

The exemplary measurement, that of LPTS, is shown in Fig. 43. The measurement of MPTS, however, is not shown, as it is analogous to the measurement of LPTS, yet using the medial tibial plateau. For more details on the measurement, I recommend consulting the original scientific paper.

* Hudek's method seems convenient for CT measurement, although it is not the only one.

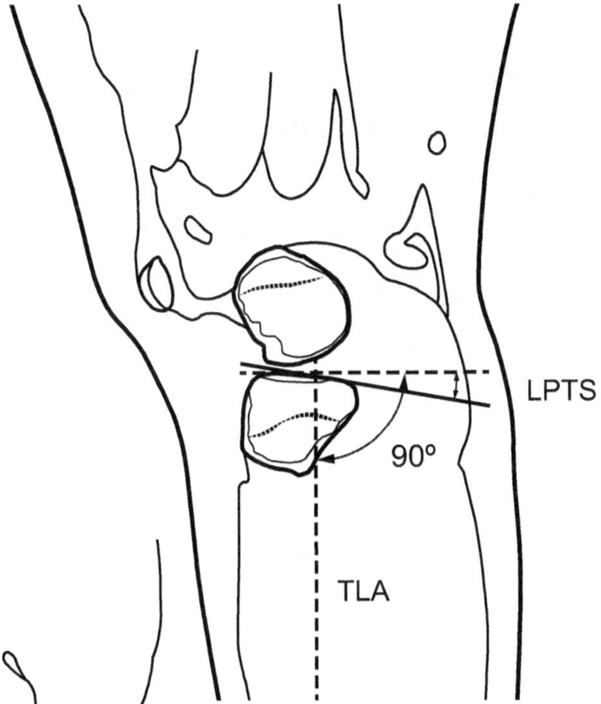

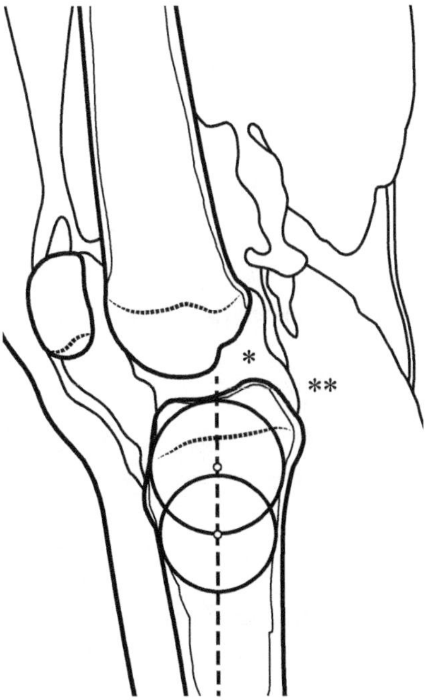

* ....eminentia intercondylaris
** .... posterior cruciate ligament attachment
LPTS .... lateral plateau posterior tibial slope (angle)
TLA ....tibial longitudinal axis

Fig. 43. Measurement of the lateral plateau posterior tibial slope angle on sagittal CT reconstructions

The Spearman's ρ for rank correlation between the *indicator* and the *medial plateau posterior tibial slope angle* was:

$$\rho = 1 - \frac{6 \times \sum d_i^2}{n \times (n^2 - 1)} = 1 - \frac{6 \times 3945.5}{30 \times (30^2 - 1)} = 1 - \frac{23673}{30 \times (900 - 1)}$$

$$= 1 - \frac{23673}{30 \times 899} = 1 - \frac{23673}{26970} = 1 - 0.88 = \mathbf{0.12}.$$

Given $\rho < \rho c$ (.12 < .47), the Spearman's correlation was not statistically significant at < .01. The magnitude was, also, 0.12.

d_i
rank difference

MPTS
medial plateau posterior tibial slope
(angle)
(°)

n
sample size
(knees)

TT-TIM
tibial tuberosity
–tibial intercondylar midpoint distance
(the indicator)
(mm)

n	Relaxation		Ranks		d_i	d_i^2
	TT-TIM	*MPTS*	*TT-TIM*	*MPTS*		
1	16	10.4	25	30	−5	25
2	14	0.8	14	2	12	144
3	12	5.7	5.5	22	−16.5	272.25
4	13	5.8	8.5	23	−14.5	210.25
5	18	1.1	28	4	24	576
6	15	2.5	20.5	10	10.5	110.25
7	13	0.9	8.5	3	5.5	30.25
8	14	3.5	14	14	0	0
9	11	1.4	3.5	6	−2.5	6.25
10	15	6.8	20.5	25	−4.5	20.25
11	14	4.6	14	20	−6	36
12	10	2.9	1.5	12	−10.5	110.25
13	15	6.5	20.5	24	−3.5	12.25
14	14	7.9	14	28	−14	196
15	11	2.9	3.5	12	−8.5	72.25
16	10	1.7	1.5	8	−6.5	42.25
17	16	1.6	25	7	18	324
18	15	1.3	20.5	5	15.5	240.25
19	15	8.5	20.5	29	−8.5	72.25
20	12	7.3	5.5	27	−21.5	462.25
21	16	0.7	25	1	24	576
22	13	2.3	8.5	9	−0.5	0.25
23	19	5.3	29.5	21	8.5	72.25
24	14	4.2	14	17.5	−3.5	12.25
25	13	4.4	8.5	19	−10.5	110.25
26	14	4.1	14	15.5	−1.5	2.25
27	14	2.9	14	12	2	4
28	15	4.2	20.5	17.5	3	9
29	17	7	27	26	1	1
30	19	4.1	29.5	15.5	14	196
Σd_i^2 =						**3945.5**

Given T > Tc (42 > 15, n = 15), the *medial plateau posterior tibial slope* (*angle*) between negatives and positives was *not statistically significant* at < .01.

The magnitude was:

d = W / S = – 36 / 120 = **– 0.30**.

– / +
negatives and positives

d
difference

| d |
absolute difference

MPTS
medial plateau posterior tibial slope
angle
(°)

n
sample size
(participants)

T
smaller sum of W– and W+ ranks

W
sum of signed ranks of difference

n			MPTS		Ranks	Signed ranks	W−	W+
	–	+	*d*	|*d*|				
1	0.8	10.4	−9.6	9.6	15	−15	−15	8.5
2	5.7	5.8	−0.1	0.1	1	−1	−1	5.5
3	2.5	1.1	1.4	1.4	8.5	8.5	−12	2.5
4	0.9	3.5	−2.6	2.6	12	−12	−14	10
5	1.4	6.8	−5.4	5.4	14	−14	−11	2.5
6	2.9	4.6	−1.7	1.7	11	−11	−8.5	13
7	6.5	7.9	−1.4	1.4	8.5	−8.5	−5.5	
8	2.9	1.7	1.2	1.2	5.5	5.5	−4	
9	1.6	1.3	0.3	0.3	2.5	2.5	−7	
10	7.3	8.5	−1.2	1.2	5.5	−5.5		
11	2.3	0.7	1.6	1.6	10	10		
12	4.2	5.3	−1.1	1.1	4	−4		
13	4.4	4.1	0.3	0.3	2.5	2.5		
14	2.9	4.2	−1.3	1.3	7	−7		
15	7	4.1	2.9	2.9	13	13		
120						−36	−78	**42**

The Spearman's ρ for rank correlation between the *indicator* and the *lateral plateau posterior tibial slope* (*angle*) was:

$$\rho = 1 - \frac{6 \times \sum d_i^2}{n \times (n^2 - 1)} = 1 - \frac{6 \times 3470}{30 \times (30^2 - 1)} = 1 - \frac{20820}{30 \times (900 - 1)}$$

$$= 1 - \frac{20820}{30 \times 899} = 1 - \frac{20820}{26970} = 1 - 0.77 = \mathbf{0.23}.$$

Given $\rho < \rho c$ (.23 < .47), the Spearman's correlation was not statistically significant at < .01. The magnitude was, also, 0.23.

d_i
rank difference

LPTS
lateral plateau posterior tibial slope
(angle)
(°)

n
sample size
(knees)

TT-TIM
tibial tuberosity
–tibial intercondylar midpoint distance
(the indicator)
(mm)

n	Relaxation		Ranks		d_i	d_i^2
	TT-TIM	*LPTS*	*TT-TIM*	*LPTS*		
1	16	6.7	25	28	–3	9
2	14	4.7	14	25	–11	121
3	12	5.5	5.5	27	–21.5	462.25
4	13	4.6	8.5	24	–15.5	240.25
5	18	4.9	28	26	2	4
6	15	1.3	20.5	7	13.5	182.25
7	13	2.4	8.5	16	–7.5	56.25
8	14	1.0	14	3	11	121
9	11	2.6	3.5	17.5	–14	196
10	15	2.3	20.5	14	6.5	42.25
11	14	1.5	14	10	4	16
12	10	3.6	1.5	22	–20.5	420.25
13	15	1.2	20.5	6	14.5	210.25
14	14	2.1	14	12	2	4
15	11	1.6	3.5	11	–7.5	56.25
16	10	1.0	1.5	3	–1.5	2.25
17	16	7.4	25	29	–4	16
18	15	1.4	20.5	8.5	12	144
19	15	3.3	20.5	20	0.5	0.25
20	12	2.9	5.5	19	–13.5	182.25
21	16	3.4	25	21	4	16
22	13	2.3	8.5	14	–5.5	30.25
23	19	7.5	29.5	30	–0.5	0.25
24	14	4.5	14	23	–9	81
25	13	1.1	8.5	5	3.5	12.25
26	14	1.4	14	8.5	5.5	30.25
27	14	1.0	14	3	11	121
28	15	0.9	20.5	1	19.5	380.25
29	17	2.3	27	14	13	169
30	19	2.6	29.5	17.5	12	144
$\Sigma d_i^2 =$						**3470**

Given T > Tc (54.5 > 15, n = 15), the *lateral plateau posterior tibial slope* (*angle*) between negatives and positives was *not statistically significant* at < .01.

The magnitude was:

d = W / S = – 11 / 120 = **– 0.09**.

– / +
negatives and positives

d
difference

| d |
absolute difference

LPTS
lateral plateau posterior tibial slope
(angle)
(°)

n
sample size
(participants)

T
smaller sum of W– and W+ ranks

W
sum of signed ranks of difference

n	LPTS				Ranks	Signed ranks	W−	W+
	−	+	*d*	|*d*|				
1	4.7	6.7	−2	2	11	−11	−11	7.5
2	5.5	4.6	0.9	0.9	7.5	7.5	−14	10
3	1.3	4.9	−3.6	3.6	14	−14	−7.5	3
4	2.4	1	1.4	1.4	10	10	−5	12
5	2.6	2.3	0.3	0.3	3	3	−9	6
6	3.6	1.5	2.1	2.1	12	12	−13	15
7	1.2	2.1	−0.9	0.9	7.5	−7.5	−3	1
8	1.6	1	0.6	0.6	6	6	−3	
9	7.4	1.4	6	6	15	15		
10	2.9	3.3	−0.4	0.4	5	−5		
11	2.3	3.4	−1.1	1.1	9	−9		
12	4.5	7.5	−3	3	13	−13		
13	1.1	1.4	−0.3	0.3	3	−3		
14	1	0.9	0.1	0.1	1	1		
15	2.3	2.6	−0.3	0.3	3	−3		
120						−11	−65.5	**54.5**

The Spearman's ρ for rank correlation between the *indicator* and *age* was:

$$\rho = 1 - \frac{6 \times \sum d_i^2}{n \times (n^2 - 1)} = 1 - \frac{6 \times 4136}{30 \times (30^2 - 1)} = 1 - \frac{24816}{30 \times (900 - 1)}$$

$$= 1 - \frac{24816}{30 \times 899} = 1 - \frac{24816}{26970} = 1 - 0.92 = \mathbf{0.08}.$$

Given $\rho < \rho c$ (.08 < .47), the Spearman's correlation was not statistically significant at < .01. The magnitude was, also, 0.08.

Due to natural pairs, the negatives and the positives had the same age of the participant they belonged to (*zero* differences for all pairs in Wilcoxon signed-rank test). Therefore, the confounding effect of age to the condition was excluded.

d_i
rank difference

n
sample size
(knees)

TT–TIM
tibial tuberosity
–tibial intercondylar midpoint distance
(the indicator)
(mm)

n	Relaxation		Ranks		d_i	d_i^2
	TT-TIM	*Age*	*TT-TIM*	*Age*		
1	16	15	25	5.5	19.5	380.25
2	14	15	14	5.5	8.5	72.25
3	12	15	5.5	5.5	0	0
4	13	15	8.5	5.5	3	9
5	18	16	28	9.5	18.5	342.25
6	15	16	20.5	9.5	11	121
7	13	17	8.5	12.5	−4	16
8	14	17	14	12.5	1.5	2.25
9	11	22	3.5	20.5	−17	289
10	15	22	20.5	20.5	0	0
11	14	15	14	5.5	8.5	72.25
12	10	15	1.5	5.5	−4	16
13	15	29	20.5	27.5	−7	49
14	14	29	14	27.5	−13.5	182.25
15	11	23	3.5	23.5	−20	400
16	10	23	1.5	23.5	−22	484
17	16	22	25	20.5	4.5	20.25
18	15	22	20.5	20.5	0	0
19	15	14	20.5	1.5	19	361
20	12	14	5.5	1.5	4	16
21	16	17	25	12.5	12.5	156.25
22	13	17	8.5	12.5	−4	16
23	19	24	29.5	25.5	4	16
24	14	24	14	25.5	−11.5	132.25
25	13	33	8.5	29.5	−21	441
26	14	33	14	29.5	−15.5	240.25
27	14	18	14	16.5	−2.5	6.25
28	15	18	20.5	16.5	4	16
29	17	18	27	16.5	10.5	110.25
30	19	18	29.5	16.5	13	169
$\Sigma d_i^2 =$						**4136**

Given T > Tc (38 > 15), the *indicator* difference between *right and left body side* was *not statistically significant* at < .01.

The magnitude was:

d = W / S = 44 / 120 = **0.37**.

d
difference

| d |
absolute difference

n
sample size
(participants)

T
smaller sum of W– and W+ ranks

TT–TIM
tibial tuberosity
–tibial intercondylar midpoint distance
(the indicator)
(mm)

W
sum of signed ranks of difference

n				**TT–TIM**	**Ranks**	**Signed ranks**	**W−**	**W+**
	Right	***Left***	***d***	***|d|***				
1	16	14	2	2	8.5	8.5	−4	8.5
2	12	13	−1	1	4	−4	−4	11
3	18	15	3	3	11	11	−13.5	13.5
4	13	14	−1	1	4	−4	−4	4
5	11	15	−4	4	13.5	−13.5	−4	4
6	14	10	4	4	13.5	13.5	−8.5	4
7	15	14	1	1	4	4		11
8	11	10	1	1	4	4		11
9	16	15	1	1	4	4		15
10	15	12	3	3	11	11		
11	16	13	3	3	11	11		
12	19	14	5	5	15	15		
13	13	14	−1	1	4	−4		
14	14	15	−1	1	4	−4		
15	17	19	−2	2	8.5	−8.5		
120						44	**−38**	82

Given T > Tc (11 > 5, n = 11), the *indicator* difference between *males and females* was *not statistically significant* at < .01.

However, the magnitude was:

d = W / S = 44 / 72 = **0.61**.

Therefore, the confounding effect of sex to the indicator was *medium*, but the sample size (n = 11) was still too small to statistically confirm it. The knees were matched by *age* and *body side*. Yet, the sample is smaller because Wilcoxon signed-rank test works only with pairs, and there were only *six* male knee pairs in the sample.

Each participant, regardless of sex, had a negative and a positive knee. So, the sex could not have had the confounding effect to the *condition*.

For those who would want to exclude this possibility utilizing statistics rather than logic, a *2x2 frequency table* (males: 6(–), 6(+), females: 9(–), 9(+), with marginal totals of 12 and 18 for sex, as well as 15 and 15 for the condition) would give P = 1.00 using *Fischer's exact test*. For more about this test, *see*, for example: Altman, 1999, pp. 253–7.

†
excluded (zero) ranks

d
difference

| d |
absolute difference

n
sample size (participants)

T
smaller sum of W– and W+ ranks

TT–TIM
tibial tuberosity –tibial intercondylar midpoint distance (the indicator) (mm)

W
sum of signed ranks of difference

n	TT–TIM				**Ranks**	**Signed ranks**	**W−**	**W+**
	Male	***Female***	***d***	$|d|$				
1	16	12	4	4	7	7	−9.5	7
2	14	13	1	1	1.5	1.5	−1.5	1.5
3	13	18	−5	5	9.5	−9.5		9.5
4	14	15	−1	1	1.5	−1.5		3
5	16	11	5	5	9.5	9.5		4.5
6†	15	15	0	—	—	—		11
7	16	14	2	2	3	3		7
8	13	10	3	3	4.5	4.5		4.5
9	19	11	8	8	11	11		7
10	14	10	4	4	7	7		
11	17	14	3	3	4.5	4.5		
12	19	15	4	4	7	7		
72						44	**−11**	55

After the relationships of interest were measured, a *magnitude plot* was drawn (Fig. 44). It was a square with a horizontal coordinate, the *magnitude*, the vertical coordinate, the *relationship of interest*, along with the *zero midline*. The *left* half of the square referred to the *indicator*, and the *right* to the *condition*. For both, an area between 0.5 magnitude on each side represented a *theoretical zone* with its borders, the *theoretical limits*. A magnitude found *inside* the theoretical limits, in the theoretical zone, had a *theoretical* importance, and its further clinical research should be minimized, if not aborted. The relationships of interest crossing the theoretical limits had at least some *practical* importance, and its further clinical research should be promoted.*

* As explained earlier in the text, for *correlations*, r ≥ .50 represents a *large* effect whereas for *differences*, on the contrary, d ≥ .80 represents a *large* effect. In both cases, however, .50 would represent a trade-off for an effect either *medium* or *large*, in other words one having a size *sufficient enough* to be of some practical merit. Therefore, in this booklet, an effect of ≥ .50 for a relationship of interest, be it correlation or difference in nature, represented an effect having enough *practical* value to be worthy of further scientific investigation in the patellofemoral stability field. Similar to many such categorizations, this one is also arbitrary, yet intuitive and, first and foremost, *pragmatic*. A great Croatian phrase suits this scenario as a glove: 'tko je jači, taj kvači', meaning the stronger calls the shots.

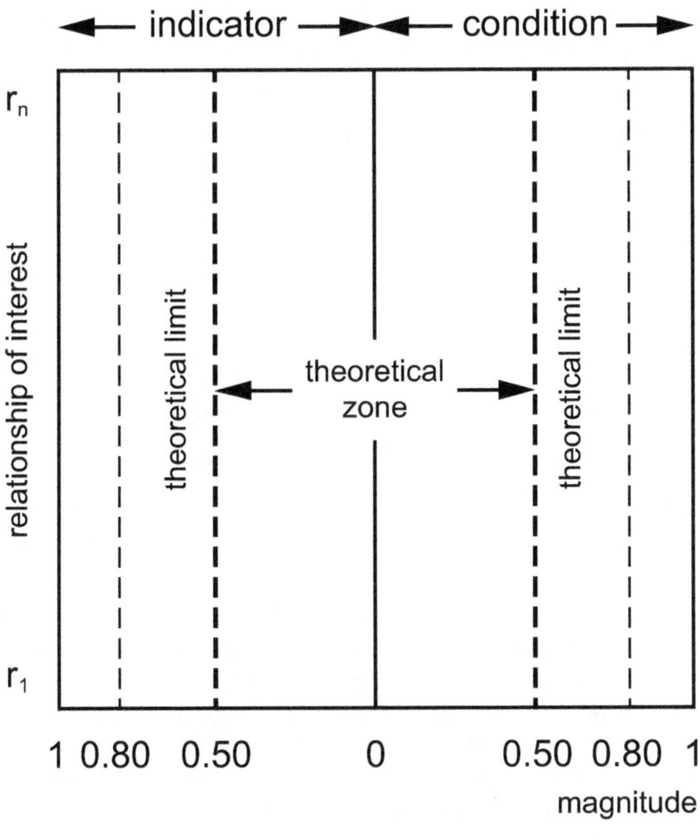

Fig. 44. Construction of the magnitude plot (relationship of interest *versus* the magnitude of that relationship)

The magnitude plot in Fig. 45 clearly shows most of the effects of external confounders to either the indicator or the condition are in the *theoretical* zone (between the inner *dashed* lines), with the exception of *sex*, exhibiting a somewhat practically important effect to the indicator (TT-TIM distance), and *FTD*, exhibiting a somewhat practically important effect to the condition (recurrent patellar dislocations), at least with regard to Caucasians. This means that if the indicator would be able to sort out the positives, it should have a *sex-split cut-off.* This, however, needs to be defined in a larger study with equal number of healthy male and female knees.

Reporting magnitudes in the field is very rare.* It was elaborated earlier that magnitudes tend to shrink when increasing the sample size. Though true, their **ranking** should remain the same. Before dealing with this in more detail, however, we shall first test the main relationship of interest in this small CT study, that between the indicator and the condition.

* Numerous studies in the evergrowing scientific literature are comparing different indicators and bone rotation angles whilst testing a plethora of different hypotheses, yet rarely reporting the sizes of the effects under investigation. Not only is this producing evidence of negligible practical importance, but is also reiterating a significant noise in this scientific field. One of the goals of this book is to highlight the utmost importance of reporting the magnitudes of different effects in a scientific paper. This is the first thing to be reported, not statistical significance as it declutters our perspective, and helps us see more clearly which relationships are worthy of further research. Therefore, it might be a good idea to do a pilot study to find these practically important relations *before* undertaking a full-blown clinical trial. This small CT study, however, cannot be considered a pilot study *per se* since the paper using much larger sample size has been published beforehand. It is, rather, an *illustrative* study, used to depict the most important topical aspects.

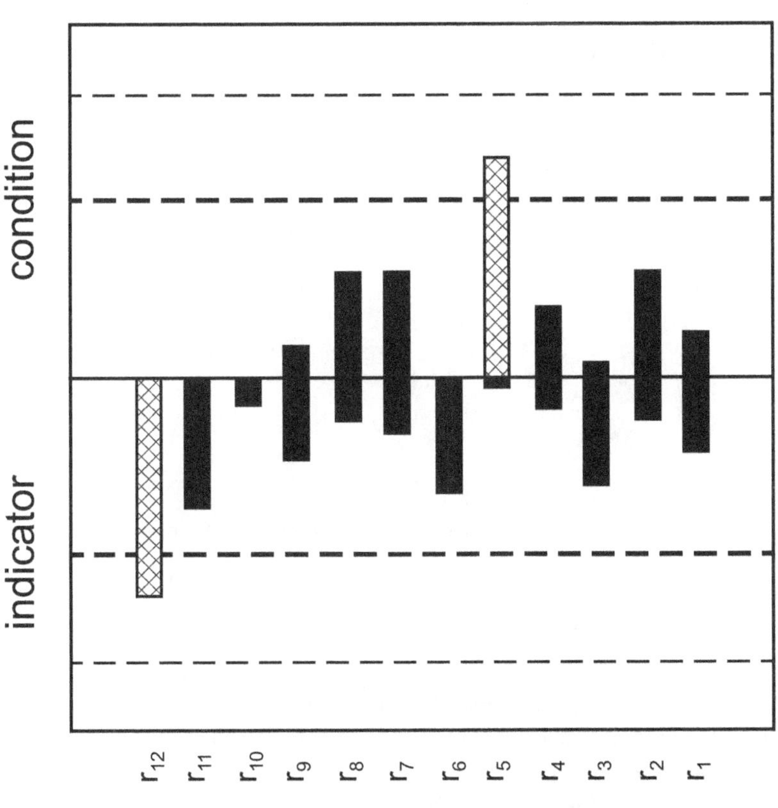

r_1 .... femoral rotation
r_2 .... tibial rotation
r_3 .... knee rotation
r_4 .... tibial torsion (at the level of the tibial tuberosity)
r_5 .... sulcus angle (femoral trochlear dysplasia)
r_6 .... extension angle (flexion–extension of the knee)
r_7 .... joint line convergence angle (varus–valgus deformity)
r_8 .... medial plateau posterior tibial slope (angle)
r_9 .... lateral plateau posterior tibial slope (angle)
r_{10} .... age
r_{11} .... body side
r_{12} .... sex

Fig. 45. Magnitude plot of external confounders with regard to the indicator–condition relationship

Given $T < Tc$ ($12 < 15$, $n = 15$), the *indicator* difference between *negatives and positives* was *statistically significant* at $< .01$.

The magnitude was:

$d = W / S = -96 / 120 = \mathbf{-0.80}$ *

Adequate statistical power protects against rejecting a *true* difference ('type II error'). The power is calculated precisely because one needs to avoid type II error. Although the sample in this small CT study was underpowered, the main relationship of interest was statistically significant and, therefore, there was no type II error.

–/+ negatives and positives	T smaller sum of W– and W+ ranks
d difference	TT–TIM tibial tuberosity –tibial intercondylar midpoint distance (the indicator) (mm)
| d | absolute difference	
n sample size (participants)	W sum of signed ranks of difference

* The fact the asymptomatic knees of patients diagnosed with unilateral patellofemoral misalignment had significantly *less* tibial tuberosity lateralization that their symptomatic knees has been known for a long time (*see*, for example, Jones *et al.*, 1995).

n	TT–TIM				Ranks	Signed ranks	W−	W+
	−	+	*d*	|*d*|				
1	14	16	−2	2	8.5	−8.5	−8.5	4
2	12	13	−1	1	4	−4	−4	4
3	15	18	−3	3	11	−11	−11	4
4	13	14	−1	1	4	−4	−4	
5	11	15	−4	4	13.5	−13.5	−13.5	
6	10	14	−4	4	13.5	−13.5	−13.5	
7	15	14	1	1	4	4	−11	
8	11	10	1	1	4	4	−11	
9	16	15	1	1	4	4	−15	
10	12	15	−3	3	11	−11	−4	
11	13	16	−3	3	11	−11	−4	
12	14	19	−5	5	15	−15	−8.5	
13	13	14	−1	1	4	−4		
14	14	15	−1	1	4	−4		
15	17	19	−2	2	8.5	−8.5		
120	200	227				−96	−108	**12**

Now, the indicator, the TT-TIM distance, is in the focus of this booklet. Therefore, it would be interesting to see how the magnitudes of relationships involving the indicator would change with *increase* of the sample size.

Should one compare the magnitudes of the relationships of external confounders and the indicator obtained from this small CT study to that from a larger, previously published CT study,* one could see most magnitudes ***decreased*, especially the largest**. Yet, interestingly, their **ranking remained the same**: the important ones were still important, and those not important were still not important. Therefore, the magnitudes decreased in their *absolute* values, but their *interpretations* were identical. This could be quite nicely described by the old Croatian proverb: 'nije šija nego vrat' (literally: 'it's not the nape but the neck'). The more it changes, the more it stays the same (on the interpretational level, at least).**

* Nizić D, Šimunović M, Pavliša G, Jelić M. Tibial tuberosity–tibial intercondylar midpoint distance measured on computed tomography scanner is not biased during knee rotation and could be clinically more relevant than current measurement systems. *Int Orthop.* 2021;45(4):959–70. DOI: 10.1007/s00264-020-04820-6.

** Once again, the *deflation* of magnitudes with increasing sample size is a known and serious problem in biostatistics. *All* of the techniques of calculating the magnitudes depend on the sample size. If solved, it could enable a much more accurate estimation of the effect size even with small samples, which would be a revolution in its own right.

Relationship	Magnitudes			
	Small CT study		*Large CT study*	
Important	**Exact**	**Absolute rounded**	**Exact**	**Absolute rounded**
TT-TIM−/+	−.80	.8	−.48	.5
Sex	.67	.7	.48	.5
Not important				
Body side	.37	.4	.20	.2
EA	−.33	.3	?	?
KR / FR-TR	.31	.3	.15	.2
LPTS	.25	.3	?	?
FR	.21	.2	.15	.2
JLCA	.16	.2	?	?
MPTS	.12	.1	?	?
TR	.10	.1	.07	.1
TITO / FTR	.09	.1	.10	.1
Age	.08	.1	−.13	.1
SA (FTD)	−.03	0	.12	.1

EA, extension angle; FR, femoral rotation (angle); JLCA, joint line convergence angle; KR, knee rotation (angle) (FR-TR is its equivalent in the large CT study); LPTS, lateral plateau posterior tibial slope (angle); MPTS, medial plateau posterior tibial slope (angle); SA, sulcus angle (defining FTD, femoral trochlear dysplasia); TITO, tibial torsion (angle) (at the level of the tibial tuberosity) (FTR is its equivalent in the large CT study); TR, tibial rotation (angle); TT-TIM, tibial tuberosity–tibial intercondylar midpoint (distance)

As mentioned earlier in this booklet, cut-offs are mostly *arbitrary*. Yet, this is not entirely true. A test **does** have its **true** cut-off, a single value called the **population mean**. However, it is **unknown**, and there is no way of knowing it. One could know it only after one has measured the indicator in the whole population. Therefore, TT-TIM's true cut-off is its population mean **one does not and cannot know**. However, although one does not know that exact number it does not mean it does not exist. For practical purposes in orthopedic surgery, one needs to have some kind of a cut-off to guide the decion-making proccess. Many are using *receiver operating characteristic* (ROC) *curves* to define a cut-off (Fig. 46). The ROC curve is a ratio of how much a test lies, *false positive rate* (FPR), as opposed to how much it tells the truth, *true positive rate* (TPR) (note it only deals with *positives*!). It was invented to see if a test A is 'better' (lies less) than test B *without the need to know the true cut-off* (which is impossible to know anyway). It is a cunning invention, but it will not help you in orthopedic practice—where one actually *needs* a practical cut-off—when the mere purpose of the curve was to **evade** defining the true cut-off. Unfortunately, with time, one reinforced the idea **any** value could be a cut-off and you just have to pick it from the curve at your own convenience, suggesting numerous ways to define it. The whole idea of endless cut-offs, however, is **not correct**. No matter how many complicated formulas mathematicians may derive, nothing can change the truth: **a test has a true cut-off, the population mean, and there is no way of knowing it**. Instead, use what is *good enough* for clinical practice!

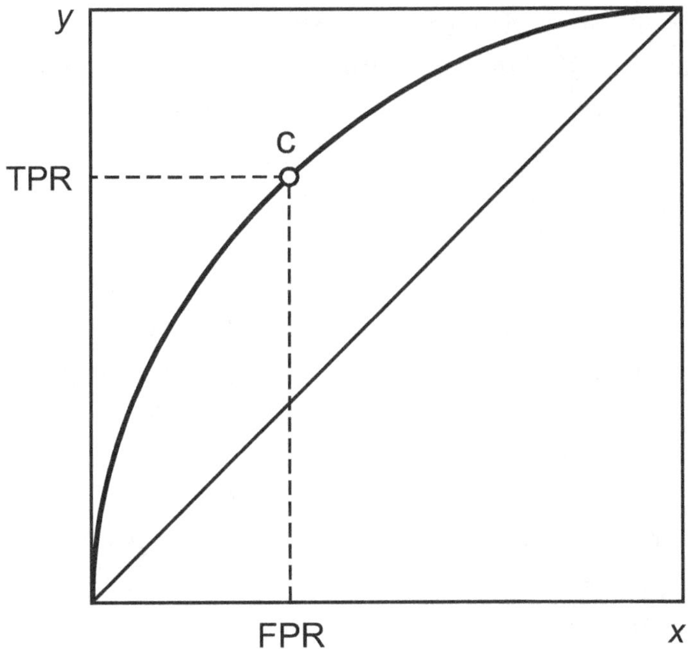

c................ cut-off
FPR .... false positive rate
TPR .... true positive rate

Fig. 46. Defining the cut-off using the receiver operating characteristic curve

But—what happens in that very clinical practice? The answer to this question is quintessential if one wants to understand what constitues an adequate diagnostic performance of the indicator.

In clinical setting, an orthopedic surgeon performs a clinical examination, and, if a patient reports several patellar dislocations without previous trauma, the patient undergoes an imaging test (say, TT-TIM distance) to see if the underlying cause of patellar instability might be the frontal misalignment. Therefore, in terms of testing, an orthopedic surgeon performs a *screening* test whereas the indicator is a *diagnostic* (imaging) *test*. Screening tests typically have *higher sensitivity* (they are better in recognizing *positives*) whereas diagnostic tests typically have *higher specificity* (they are better in recognizing *negatives*). The role of an orthopedic surgeon is to *include* the ill, and the role of the indicator is to *exclude* the healthy (so they can evade unneccessary therapy, above all potentially harmful surgical procedures). The **diagnostic synergy** of an orthopedic surgeon and the indicator should produce sensitivity and specificity of *around 80%* (Fig. 47). Therefore, **one must not forget the indicator is measured in the *clinical* setting, following the *clinical* examination.** In this context (and context is everything!), the sensitivity of the indicator is, therefore, **irrelevant** (though it should be *above 50%* to be called a test).*

* A test with sensitivity and specificity of 100%, mind you, represents an *ideal*, and is not achievable in biosystems. Also, anything *below* 50% is *guessing*. This is another reason against cherry-picking a high specificity cut-off from the ROC curve, as it automatically *lowers* sensitivity under 50%.

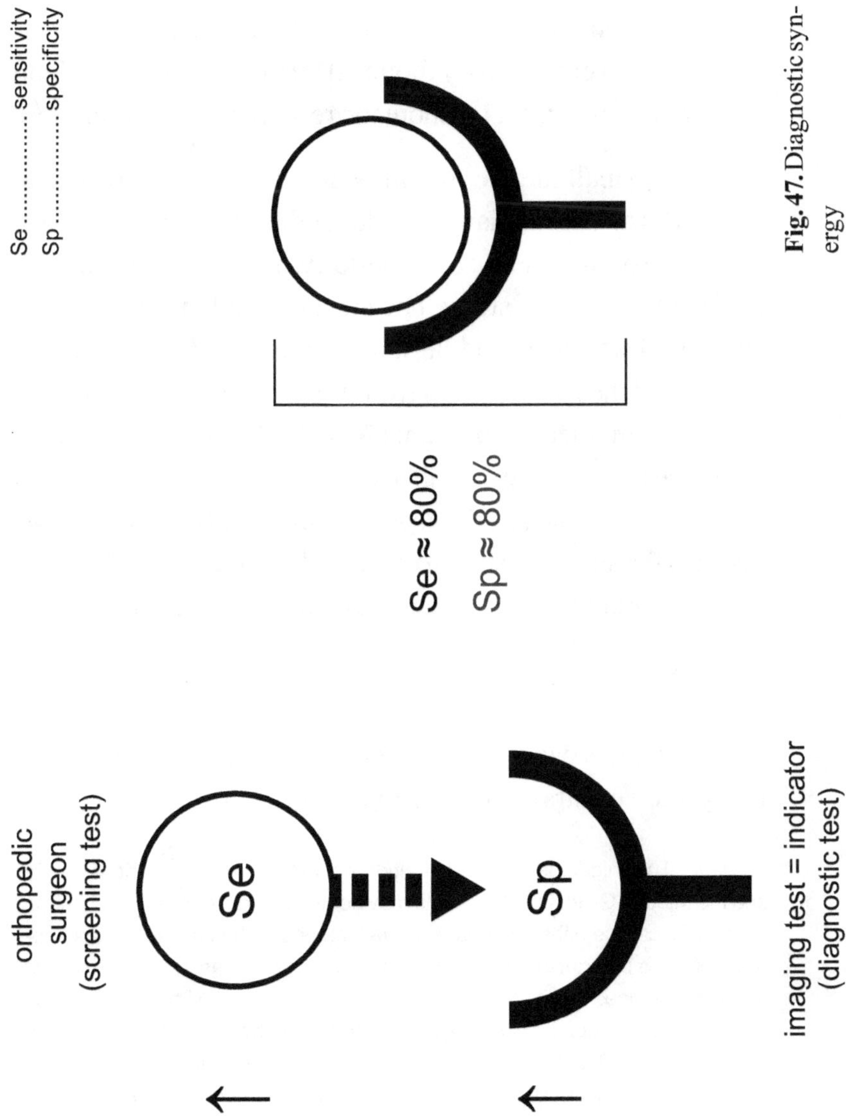

Fig. 47. Diagnostic synergy

Yet, there is a bit of a problem here: the cut-off must not be cherry-picked from the ROC curve to simply reflect high specificity (as is often erroneously thought) but, rather, it should lend itself to the researcher (without the researcher's intervention).

Due to the small sample size, the safest bet one has is to look at the **median**. The median is not dependent on extreme values, and hence on symmetric distribution which cannot be guaranteed in this small CT study. The median was **14 mm**. Since the number 14 was in the middle, it was neither left (–) nor right (+), and should thus be *excluded* from further calculus.* A total of 23 pairs remained, 17 of them (74%; 17/23) counting according to the truth (so the overall accuracy of the test was **74%**). If number 13 is considered a *negative*, and number 15 a *positive*, one gets the situation shown in the table on the right. Counting the four possible pairs of outcomes, one can see the following:

+/+=**9** –/+=**4** +/–=**2** –/–=**8.**

From this, it is easy to construct a *2x2 frequency table* with four possible pairs of outcomes (+/+, –/+, +/–, and –/–).

* The middle is the *third* position because one has the right, the left and the middle. Given that the middle may be neither right nor left, which means it, actually, can be either, it should not be included in the calculus. It is a separate entity. To be right or left, you first have to be neither as this is the only way to have a choice. The choice itself may become evident with *time*, after, say, a 3-month follow-up. It is likewise interesting to note here that the overall accuracy of the TT-TG distance is 69% (AUC=.69; 95%CI = .60, .79) (Moya-Angeler *et al.*, 2022). In addition, having a *unitless* ratio such as *TT-TG distance/trochlear dysplasia index* (with 1.88 cut-off) as proposed by Moya-Angeler *et al.* instead of a millimeter distance is not practical from a surgical viewpoint as the desired amount of millimeter correction remains unknown.

Truth	Indicator	Truth	Indicator
–	*TT-TIM*	+	*TT-TIM*
~~14~~		16	+
12	–	13	–
15	+	18	+
13	–	~~14~~	
11	–	15	+
10	–	~~14~~	
15	+	~~14~~	
11	–	10	–
16	+	15	+
12	–	15	+
13	–	16	+
~~14~~		19	+
13	–	~~14~~	
~~14~~		15	+
17	+	19	+

'–', negatives; '+', positives; TT-TIM, tibial tuberosity–tibial intercondylar midpoint (distance)

The 2x2 frequency table consists of **outer**, and **inner** counts, former being the **totals**. Clearly, the outer counts are very close to one another (11 and 13, 12 and 10) implying the indicator (TT-TIM distance) sorts quite similar to the truth.*

With a 14 mm cut-off, the indicator (TT-TIM distance) had a sensitivity of **69% (9/13)** and specificity of **80% (8/10)**. This would mean the values **≤ 13 mm** are **negatives** and need no therapy, the values ≥ **15 mm** are **positives** and need therapy whereas the value of **14 mm** is **neutral** and needs a 3-month follow-up.

On closer inspection of 95% confidence intervals, one could notice sensitivity and specificity might be even *higher* in population, as high as *90% or more*, especially the latter, which was the main goal to begin with. No cherry-picking either—instead, the plane and simple median was used as the cut-off between the negatives and the positives.**

But all of this is valid **only** if one completely ignores the sex bias treating males and females as having the same cut-off. Yet, as one could have learned earlier in this booklet, this is not true: **males have larger cut-offs**. Hence, it would be a gross mistake simply to ignore the influence of sex as the external confounder to the indicator. Now what?

* If one would like to test this obvious conclusion using McNemar's test for paired proportions, the results would be as following: the difference = 8.7%, 95% confidence interval: –14.5, 23.8, P = 0.69 at α = .05.

** In a perfectly symmetric distributions, of course, the mean and the median are *equal*.

TT-TIM distance		Truth	Total
> 14 mm	+	–	
+	9	2	**11**
–	4	8	**12**
Total	**13**	**10**	***23***

TT-TIM distance	Diagnostic validity
Sensitivity	**69%** (39–91)
Specificity	**80%** (44–98)
Area under the curve (AUC)	**.8** (.5–.9)
Positive likelihood ratio	**3.5** (1.0–12.6)
Negative likelihood ratio	**0.4** (0.2–0.9)
Positive predictive value	**82%** (48–98)
Negative predictive value	**67%** (35–90)

TT-TIM distance	Action
≤ **13** mm	no therapy
14 mm	3-month follow-up
≥ **15** mm	therapy

mm.................................. millimeters
TT-TIM................... tibial tuberosity–tibial intercondylar midpoint (distance)

The only way to properly answer the question of sex-split cut-offs would be to collect a *very large* sample (≈ 1,500 knees for each sex) with *equal* number of male and female healthy knee pairs of certain *ethinicity* and to report their sex means with 95% confidence intervals (or better yet: *medians*?), preferably as *narrow* as possible. It is imperative the cut-offs should be studied with regard to *different* ethnicites.

Until then, since a larger study on TT-TIM distance has been published, it might be benefitial to investigate the possible cut-offs based on its somewhat larger sample size, mostly for informative purposes. A closer look at the data reveals even with n = 25 for males and n = 82 for females, the situation has not changed much: the specificity is *still around 80%*, especially when one looks at the 95% confidence intervals: **80%** (12/15) (95% CI: 52, 96) for males and **76%** (28/37) (95% CI: 59, 88) for females whereas sensitivity has dropped a bit (males: **60%**: 26, 88 and females: **62%**: 47, 76).* Therefore, the specificity appears to hold on inspite of much higher variability in the sample, which is certainly encouraging, especially in the light of the fact TT-TIM values were *averaged* after two blinded raters performed the measurements at two-week intervals.**

* Again, if one would like to test if TT-TIM and the truth sort differently using McNemar's test for paired proportions, which they obviously should not, according to the tables on the right the results would be as following: for males, the difference = 4.0%, 95% confidence interval: –17.7, 22.5, P = 1.00, and for females, the difference = 9.8%, 95% confidence interval: –3.6, 20.8, P = 0.17 at $\alpha = .05$.

** Due to objective circumstances, the issue of *inter-rater reliability* could not be addressed in this small CT study. However, in its larger counterpart the ICC was > .80. For more on ICCs in general, *see* Shrout and Fleiss, 1979.

TT-TIM distance		**Truth**	**Total**
males > 15 mm	+	–	
+	6	3	**9**
–	4	12	**16**
Total	**10**	**15**	***25***

TT-TIM distance		**Truth**	**Total**
females > 12 mm	+	–	
+	28	9	**37**
–	17	28	**45**
Total	**45**	**37**	***82***

TT-TIM distance (males)	**Action**
≤ **14** mm	no therapy
15 mm	3-month follow-up
≥ **16** mm	therapy

TT-TIM distance (females)	**Action**
≤ **11** mm	no therapy
12 mm	3-month follow-up
≥ **13** mm	therapy

mm................................ millimeters
TT-TIM .... tibial tuberosity–
tibial intercondylar midpoint (distance)

Accuracy is the closeness of the measured value and the true value, and, more statistically, a deviation of an estimate from the true population value (Kirch *et al.*, 2008, p. 2). Accuracy and precision, however, are not the same (Kirch *et al.*, 2008, p. 1126). High precision is necessary for high accuracy, but the reverse does not hold (Kirch *et al.*, 2008, p. 1126).

To complicate the discussion on these concepts even further, precision is akin to something called *reliability*, but they are not the same either. Precision refers to consistency of *repeated results* whereas reliability refers to consistency of *measurement instrument* (Kirch *et al.*, 2008, pp. 890–1, 1249). Therefore, precision refers to the consistency of an *imaging test* whereas the reliability refers to the consistency of an *imaging instrument* (XR, CT or MRI scanner). A subtle, yet important difference! But, what does it all *really* mean?

Well, *precision* is analyzed using the measures of 'imprecision' (variance [Var], sd, and coefficient of variation [CV])* whereas *reliability* is analyzed using the measures of reliability (internal consistency reliability, test–retest reliability, and inter-rater reliability) (Kirch *et al.*, 2008, pp. 890, 1249). In majority of scientific work in this field, ICCs are used as a measure of inter-rater reliability. However, having all the

* Sds are used to compare variables with the *same* measurement unit whereas CVs are used to compare vairables with *different* measurement units (Rani, 2012, Ch4: 4.10–11). Given that all distances are expressed in the same measurement unit (millimeters), sds should be used for mutual comparison. On the other hand, Var is already included in the sd calculus.

aforementioned in mind, one has to understand high ICCs represent high reliability of an *imaging instrument* (that is indirectly evaluated by the raters), and not high precision of an imaging test *itself*, as it may be implied. If precision of an imaging test is very *high*, Var, sd and CV are very *low*. The factor further influencing the precision of a measurement instrument is the *resolution*, the smallest change of the measurement value that a measurement instrument can show (Kirch *et al.*, 2008, p. 890). The smaller the measurable change, the higher the reliability of the CT/MRI, I guess. So, to sum it all up: **the precision of the TT-TIM distance depends on its *sd* whereas the reliability of CT scanner for measurement of TT-TIM distance depends, mostly, on the *ICC*.** Since I am a single researcher in this small CT study, if I were to investigate whether CT is a reliable measurement instrument to measure TT-TIM distance, I would obviously need to circumvent inter-rater reliability and find a way to unveil the truth using test–retest reliability. In biostatistics, **test–retest reliability** is an estimation of the scale of stability over time that is measure of result congruency obtained by repeated measurement of the same objects, under the condition that there was no change in the condition of those objects (Kirch *et al.*, 2008, p. 1249). Therefore, the best I could do to test the reliability of this particular CT scanner (16-row, Siemens Medical Systems, Erlangen, Germany) for measurement of TT-TIM distance as a single researcher in this small CT study was to select the first knee from the list, and perform 15 measurements of the TT-TIM distance *on that same right knee* with each entry having a daily interval in between.

Therefore, for thirty days, I measured the TT-TIM distance every other day to try to decrease the *recall bias*. The technical parameters were: 40–55 mA, 130kV, slice thickness 2 mm of the bone (width = 1500, mean = 450) and soft-tissue window (width = 450, mean = 45).

And? What did I find? What was the reliability of this particular CT scanner for measurement of TT-TIM distance? The results are in the table on the right.

The exact values do not follow normal distribution, and median is 16.1 mm (95% CI: 15.6, 16.1). If one would take the difference between the lowest and the highest value, divide it with the lowest value and calculate the percentage, the exact reliability would be somewhat lower:

16.4 – 15.5 = 0.9 / 16.4 = 0.06 × 100% = 6%.
16.4 – 15.5 = 0.9 / 15.5 = 0.06 × 100% = 6%.
100% – 6% = **94%.**

If one should round the resulting values, it would become obvious that each time the value of the indicator was consistently the same, 16 mm. Therefore, the reliability of this CT scanner for measurement of the TT-TIM distance was **100%, provided that integers were used**.

n
number of measurements

TT–TIM
tibial tuberosity
–tibial intercondylar midpoint distance
(the indicator)
(mm)

n	Test–retest reliability in quadriceps relaxation	
	TT-TIM exact	*TT-TIM rounded*
1	15.8	16
2	15.5	16
3	15.8	16
4	16.1	16
5	16.1	16
6	15.8	16
7	15.5	16
8	16.1	16
9	16.1	16
10	15.5	16
11	16.4	16
12	16.4	16
13	16.4	16
14	15.5	16
15	16.1	16
	94%	**100%**

I would imagine original authors of an imaging test (a millimeter distance) are likely the ones to measure it in *the most precise manner*. If one should compare the sds of some of these distances as they were first reported in their original scientific papers, and case- and control group sds were averaged,* it would appear, for example, TT-TIM distance is **36% more precise** than its closest neighbour, TT-PCL distance. Given that 33.33% is approximately ⅓, could one label this difference as substantial? Most probably, yes! Other counterparts scored much worse (*see* the table on the right).**

An imaging test—let me reiterate this—must be accurate *as well as* precise! **An accurate test, yet imprecise is not fit for practical use and must be immediately abandoned regardless of any other advantages it may possess.** Precision of a test is often overlooked, although its importance cannot be overstated! If a test is not able to repeatedly put the *same* study unit into the *same* category, it is practically useless. Whether the category is true or false, however, is a matter of *accuracy*.

* Some sds were not even reported in their original scientific papers. For example, TT-MIELTI did not report its sds (Keehan *et al.*, 2019). Therefore, results from the only work on the subject currently available, that of Li *et al.*, 2024. were used. Li *et al.* also found TT-TIM distance to be *inaccurate*. On page 5, the authors show Table 3, where TT-TIM distance has the *lowest* sds, from 3.2 mm in the study group to 4.0 mm in the control group (versus 6.8 mm and 4.8 mm respectively for their favorite, the TT-TG distance). Isn't it odd the *most precise* method in the study was the *only one* to get it wrong, more so if we know high precision is necessary for high accuracy? Or is it, perhaps, it refused to validate a flawed sample design? The contradiction is what made me write this book. I, therefore, thank the authors for the impetus.

** Perhaps *imprecision* rather than knee rotation is the reason why TT-TG distance changes even without intervention (Pascual-Leone *et al.*, 2023).

Distance	Reference	Precision	
		Average sd (mm)	*Percentage (%)*
TT-TIM	Nizić *et al.*, 2021	2.8	—
TT-PCL	Seitlinger *et al.*, 2012	(4.30+3.35) / 2 = 3.8	– 36
TT-RA	Xu *et al.*, 2020	(4.41+4.24) / 2 = 4.3	– 54
TT-ME	Iseki *et al.*, 2020	4.6	– 64
TT-TG	Nizić *et al.*, 2021	6.0	– 114
TT-MIELTI	Li *et al.*, 2024	(8.4+5.3) / 2 = 6.9	– 146

sd, standard deviation; TT-ME, tibial tuberosity–midepicondyle (distance); TT-MIELTI, tibial tuberosity–mid inter-epicondyle trochlea intersection (distance); TT-PCL, tibial tuberosity–posterior cruciate ligament (distance); TT-RA, tibial tuberosity–Roman arch (distance); TT-TG, tibial tuberosity–trochlear groove (distance); TT-TIM, tibial tuberosity–tibial intercondylar midpoint (distance)

The same variable measured on different imaging modalities without intervention should give the same value. If one has measured the same variable, say distance between the relative middle of the leg/knee and the tibial tuberosity on XR and CT, the measurements should **overlap**. By comparison, the XR values of TA-GT distance from the original French paper (Goutallier *et al.*, 1978), and the CT values of TT-TIM distance (Nizić *et al.*, 2021) largely overlap.* Moreover, TA-GT distance had normative XR values between 10 and 15 mm (Dahhan *et al.*, 1981, p. 37) whereas TT-TIM distance had one sd range from 10 to 15.6 mm (Fig. 48). **This suggests TA-GT and TT-TIM measure the same variable (distance).**

Since CT values of TT-TIM distance followed a **symmetric curve**, one could use **empirical rules** to predict the extreme values of TT-TIM distance (Serdar, 1966, p. 112. Fig. 2.9.):

$$\Pr(\mu - 1\text{sd} \leq x \leq \mu + 1\text{sd}) \approx 68.27\%$$
$$\Pr(\mu - 2\text{sd} \leq x \leq \mu + 2\text{sd}) \approx 95.45\%$$
$$\Pr(\mu - 3\text{sd} \leq x \leq \mu + 3\text{sd}) \approx 99.73\%.$$

Hence, a value **below 4 mm and above 21 mm** may be a possible error as some TT-TIM values are almost unattainable (Fig. 48). Typically, the value of TT-TIM distance is a **positive integer**.

* The mean value of TT-TIM distance was 12.8±2.8 mm, with 2 sds, covering 95.45% of values, ranging from 7.2 to 18.4 mm (Nizić *et al.*, 2021). In the paper of Goutallier *et al.*, 1978, the mean value of TA-GT distance was around 13 mm ('TA-GT: la valeur moyenne est d'environ 13 mm', p. 427), ranging from 7 to 17 mm ('Les distances TA-GT pour le groupe témoin sont faibles et comprises entre 7 et 17 mm.', p. 427). In comparison, the control values for TT-TIM distance in this study (p. 163) were between 10 and 17 mm, hence rather similar (though at different sample sizes!).

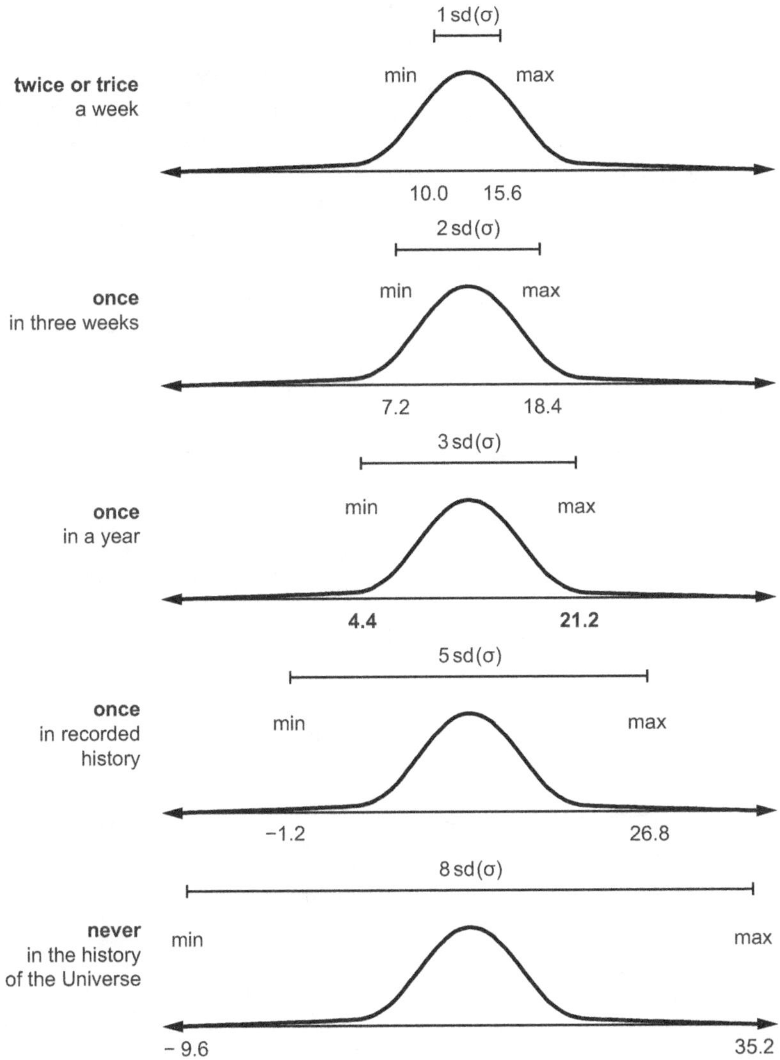

max........... maximum
min............ minimum
sd.............. standard deviation (σ)

Fig. 48. Symmetric curves of TT-TIM distance at different standard deviations (sigmas) exhibiting extremes

3

Tracking Validity and Internal Confounders

Given that the indicator was able to adequately sort out the positives, one now has to ensure it has a *tracking* validity. This simply means it is capable of tracking a therapeutic response. But, before going any further, one should ask: what *is* therapy anyway?

In broadest sense, a therapy is a *change*: a change from state A (*before* therapy) to state B (*after* therapy). In terms of this field of research, the change would be the change of *spatial position of the quadriceps insertion, the TT.* What conservative and surgical therapy alike are trying to achieve is to *medialize* the TT, in other words: to bring it *closer* to the relative middle of the knee, be it by the strengthening of the quadriceps mechanism to increase internal tibial rotation (*conservative* therapy) or physically translocating the TT from one anatomical position to another performing TT transfer (TTT) (*surgical* therapy). In both instances, TT needs to be *medialized.* According to the 'wall and ball theory', explained earlier in the text, to register the movement of the TT point, the point reflecting the relative middle of the knee, the TIM point, *must be static*, that is to say, must be on the same anatomical spot on the bone from one tibia to another, from one individual to another, regardless of anatomical variability. Using pericondylar rectangle will assure TIM is always in the middle of the proximal part of the tibia. If TT were a dynamic and TIM a static point, upon therapy, the value of the indicator, TT-TIM distance, should *decrease* (Fig. 49). Therefore, all one has to prove is that, upon changing the TT's spatial position, TT-TIM distance **decreases**.

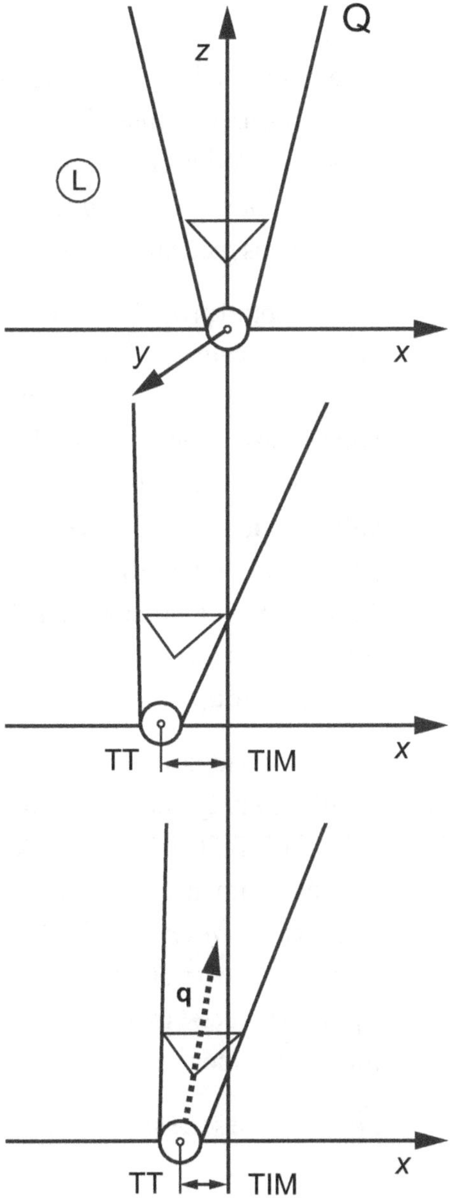

L................................ lateral
q ....quadriceps vector
Q....................... quadriceps mechanism
TT-TIM.......tibial tuberosity-tibial intercondylar midpoint (distance)
x-y-z............................ axes (of the orthogonal coordinate system)

Fig. 49. Decrease of the TT-TIM distance upon activation of the quadriceps mechanism

In this small CT study, the quadriceps mechanism was activated using MVIC. This means, upon MVIC, TT-TIM should *decrease*, and the magnitude of the effect should be *practically important.* What is more, this needs to be investigated in negatives and positives *taken together* (because each of them has a quadriceps mechanism) (Fig. 50).

If that should prove to be the case, if MVIC would actually *decrease* the value of TT-TIM distance in participants who have not undergone *any* therapy, one could reasonably hypothesize conservative therapy should *decrease* the value of TT-TIM distance in quadriceps relaxation towards the normative values, mitigating the need for surgical therapy that could be performed only with more severe cases. In other words: **TT-TIM distance measured *after* therapy could be a *benchmark* of therapy success, either in conservative or surgical therapeutic approaches.**

Given that negatives and positives are taken together, in this small CT study one suddendly has two groups at hand, each n = 30: the TT-TIM distance in knees *before* MVIC (with quadriceps mechanism relaxation), and the TT-TIM distance in those same knees *after* MVIC. The 100% increase of sample size, from n = 15 to n = 30 *increases* statistical power of the Wilcoxon signed-rank test in the study around 2.7 times, from .18 to .48 for magnitudes > .5 at $\alpha = .01$.

So, what does the statistical analysis show?

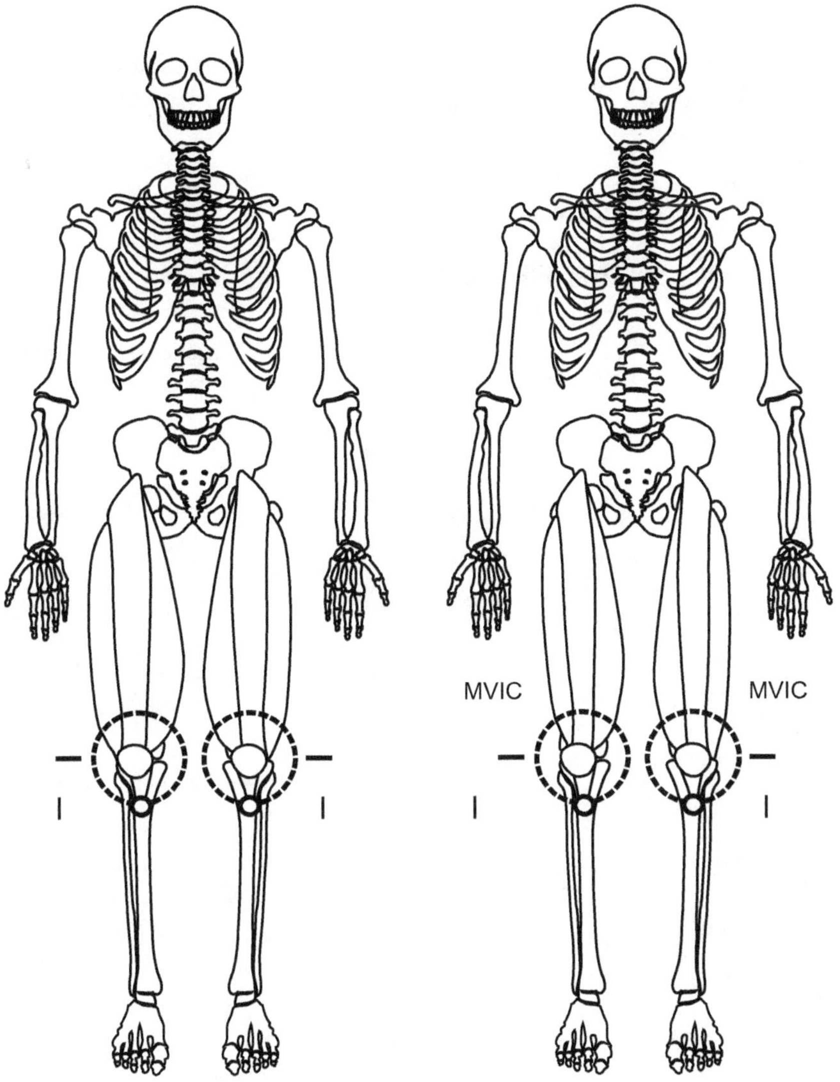

MVIC .... maximum voluntary isometric contraction
I... indicator

Fig. 50. Relaxation (*left*) and maximum voluntary isometric contraction of the quadriceps mechanism (*right*) (negative)

Given T < Tc (4.5 < 54, n = 23), the *indicator* difference between *relaxation and MVIC* was *statistically significant* at < .01.

The magnitude was:

d = W / S = 267 / 378 = **0.71**.

†
excluded (zero) ranks

d
difference

| d |
absolute difference

n
sample size

R – / +
relaxation of the quadriceps mechanism
in negatives and positives

T
smaller sum of W– and W+ ranks

TT–TIM
tibial tuberosity
–tibial intercondylar midpoint distance
(the indicator)
(mm)

MVIC – / +
maximum voluntary isometric contraction
of th quadriceps mechanism
in negatives and positives

W
sum of signed ranks of difference

n				TT–TIM	Ranks	Signed ranks	W−	W+
	R−/+	*MVIC*−/+	*d*	|*d*|				
1 †	16	16	0	—	—	—	−4.5	12
2	14	12	2	2	12	12		12
3	12	10	2	2	12	12		19
4	13	10	3	3	19	19		4.5
5	18	17	1	1	4.5	4.5		12
6 †	15	15	0	—	—	—		19
7	13	11	2	2	12	12		23
8	14	11	3	3	19	19		4.5
9 †	11	11	0	—	—	—		4.5
10 †	15	15	0	—	—	—		12
11	14	9	5	5	23	23		12
12	10	9	1	1	4.5	4.5		4.5
13 †	15	15	0	—	—	—		19
14	14	13	1	1	4.5	4.5		4.5
15	11	9	2	2	12	12		19
16	10	8	2	2	12	12		4.5
17	16	15	1	1	4.5	4.5		19
18	15	12	3	3	19	19		12
19	15	14	1	1	4.5	4.5		19
20	12	9	3	3	19	19		12
21 †	16	16	0	—	—	—		4.5
22	13	12	1	1	4.5	4.5		19
23	19	16	3	3	19	19		
24	14	15	−1	1	4.5	−4.5		
25	13	11	2	2	12	12		
26	14	11	3	3	19	19		
27 †	14	14	0	—	—	—		
28	15	13	2	2	12	12		
29	17	16	1	1	4.5	4.5		
30	19	16	3	3	19	19		
378	427	381				267	**−4.5**	271.5

Therefore, yes: TT-TIM distance *decreases* with MVIC, and the magnitude of that effect is *medium*, and statistically significant, even in the sample of this size.*

Since the TT point belongs to the dynamic quadriceps mechanism, that is to say it has an ability to change its spatial position, one should regard it as the *dynamic* point. In addition, as it belongs to the quadriceps mechanism, it is only logical the actions of the quadriceps mechanism should influence the indicator, TT-TIM distance, because, let us remember that, the TT point is a part of the indicator. This impact is, therefore, *completely logical.* It also means TT-TIM distance will most likely register the activation of the quadriceps mechanism (as was indeed proven). Likewise, the effects of internal confounders, those *within* the quadriceps mechanism to the indicator should be *theoretical* (Fig. 51).

We have studied external confounders and their influence on the indicator–condition relationship. Now, we shall embark to see the state of affairs regarding *internal* confounders.

* This a 'proof-of-concept' study. Therefore, the size of an effect is not of interest here, it need not be large. The fact that the value of the indicator, the TT-TIM distance *decreases* after MVIC is in itself the proof of the 'wall and ball theory' concept.

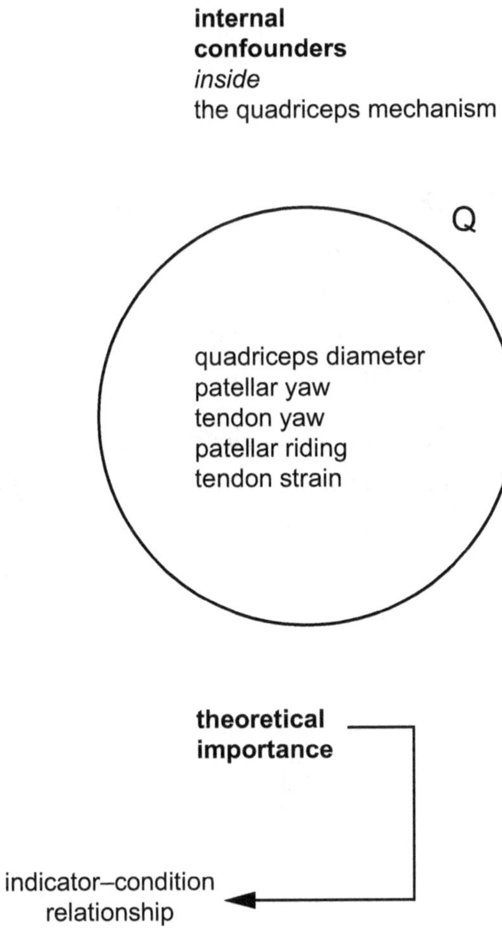

Q..... quadriceps mechanism

Fig. 51. Internal confounders to the indicator–condition relationship

Transverse diameter of the quadriceps belly (φ; Greek small letter 'phi') is a function of quadriceps belly strength: the *larger* the transverse diameter of the quadriceps belly, the *stronger* the quadriceps belly. This new parameter, φ, is reported in *centimeters*.

To ensure quadriceps belly has undergone MVIC, the value of φ was measured *6 cm above the patellar basis* in negatives and positives. Using 2-mm cuts, this means φ was measured on the 30th cranial CT image from the CT image on which the patella was no longer visible (30 × 2 mm = 60 mm = 6 cm) (the '6-cut') (Fig. 52).*

* In this small CT study, the 6 cm level was high enough in all participants who underwent CT imaging to comprise all four heads of the quadriceps muscle, that is to say: the *entire quadriceps belly.*

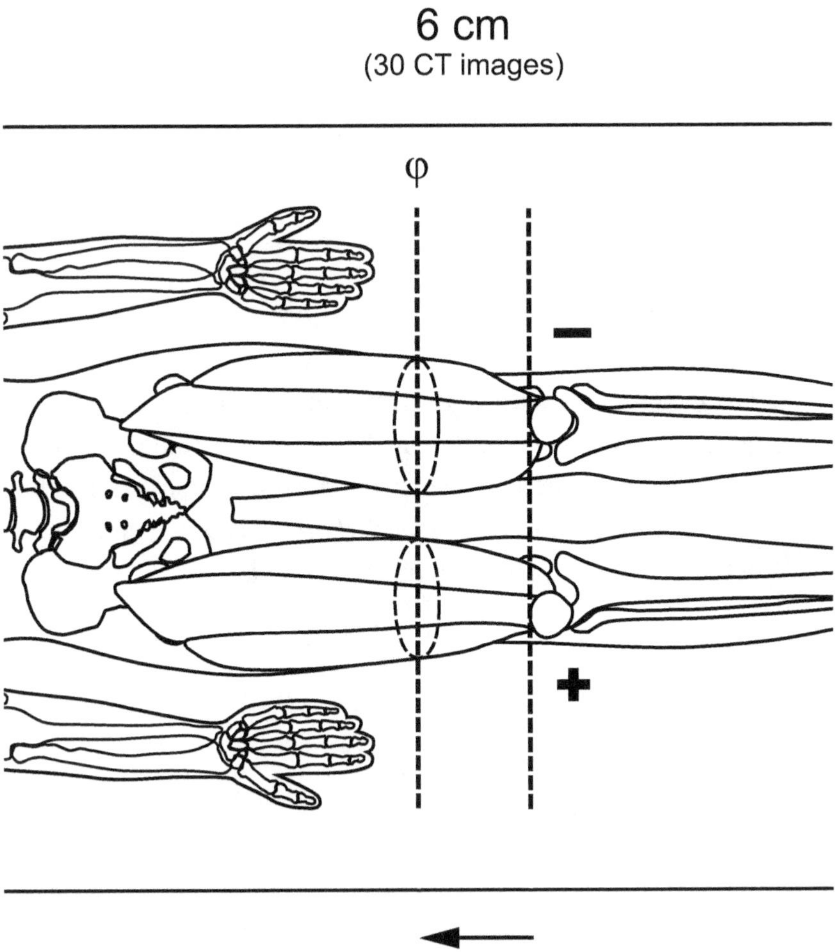

–/+ .... negatives and positives
φ ....transverse diameter of the quadriceps belly

Fig. 52. Measurement level for the transverse diameter of the quadriceps belly on supine CT imaging (the '6-cut')

The idea was to measure the transverse diameter of the *entire* quadriceps belly. Therefore, in the transverse plane, this could be easily performed by measuring the transverse distance between *two vertical lateral / medial tangents* of the quadriceps belly (disregarding the thin fibers on the sides).

The main principle is shown in Fig. 53.

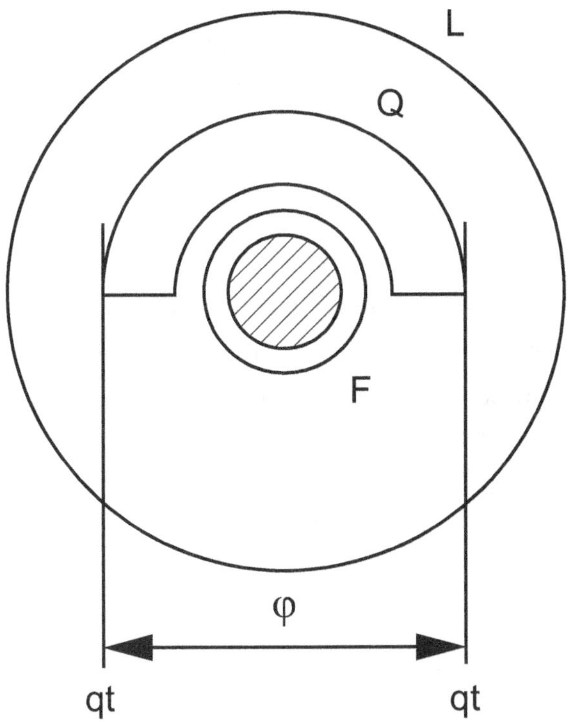

φ .... transverse diameter of the quadriceps belly
F .... femur
L.. leg
qt............... quadriceps belly tangent (lateral / medial)
Q............................ quadriceps belly

Fig. 53. Measurement of the transverse diameter of the quadriceps belly on the '6-cut' transverse CT image (*principle*)

In the transverse plane, on the '6-cut' CT image, the horizontal distance between two vertical diagonals was φ in centimeters. In this small CT study, in all thirty knees, it was a quick and easy measurement (Fig. 54).

Hence, upon MVIC, one expects the value of φ to *decrease*.

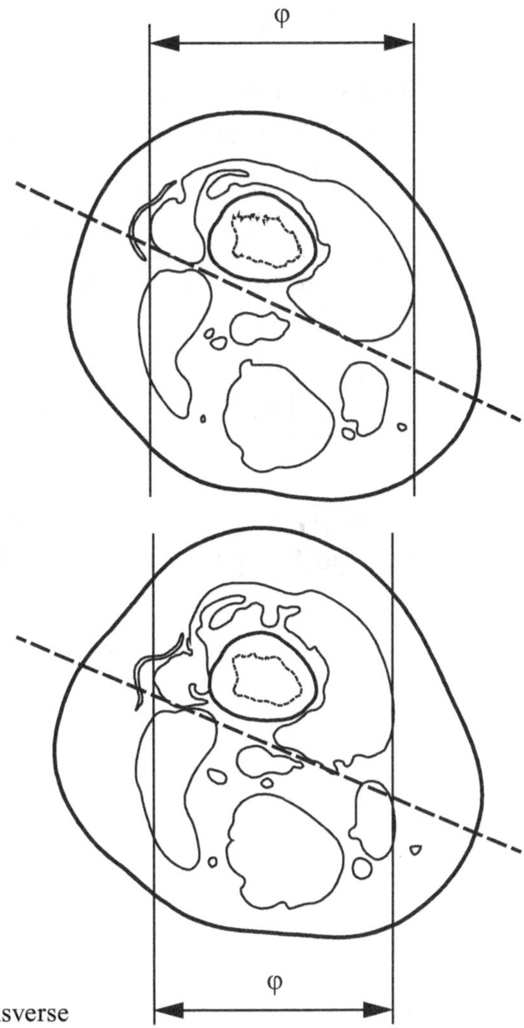

Fig. 54. Measurement of the transverse diameter of the quadriceps belly on the '6-cut' transverse CT image in relaxation (*above*) and maximum voluntary isometric contraction of the quadriceps mechanism (*below*)

The Spearman's ρ for rank correlation between the *indicator* and the *transverse diameter of the quadriceps belly* was:

$$\rho = 1 - \frac{6 \times \sum d_i^2}{n \times (n^2 - 1)} = 1 - \frac{6 \times 4016.5}{30 \times (30^2 - 1)} = 1 - \frac{24099}{30 \times (900 - 1)}$$

$$= 1 - \frac{24099}{30 \times 899} = 1 - \frac{24099}{26970} = 1 - 0.89 = \mathbf{0.11.}$$

Given $\rho < \rho c$ (.11 < .47), the Spearman's correlation was not statistically significant at < .01. The magnitude was, also, 0.11.

d_i
rank difference

φ
transverse diameter
of the quadriceps belly
in negatives and positives
(cm)

n
sample size (knees)

TT–TIM
tibial tuberosity
–tibial intercondylar midpoint distance
in negatives and positives
(the indicator)
(mm)

n	Relaxation		Ranks		d_i	d_i^2
	TT-TIM	φ	*TT-TIM*	φ		
1	16	9.53	25	18	7	49
2	14	9.34	14	14	0	0
3	12	8.21	5.5	6	−0.5	0.25
4	13	8.05	8.5	4	4.5	20.25
5	18	10.02	28	27	1	1
6	15	10.05	20.5	28	−7.5	56.25
7	13	9.96	8.5	26	−17.5	306.25
8	14	9.72	14	21	−7	49
9	11	10.06	3.5	29	−25.5	650.25
10	15	9.25	20.5	12	8.5	72.25
11	14	9.30	14	13	1	1
12	10	9.84	1.5	23	−21.5	462.25
13	15	8.99	20.5	10	10.5	110.25
14	14	8.60	14	8	6	36
15	11	9.46	3.5	16	−12.5	156.25
16	10	8.39	1.5	7	−5.5	30.25
17	16	9.48	25	17	8	64
18	15	9.66	20.5	19	1.5	2.25
19	15	8.00	20.5	3	17.5	306.25
20	12	8.18	5.5	5	0.5	0.25
21	16	9.73	25	22	3	9
22	13	10.33	8.5	30	−21.5	462.25
23	19	9.70	29.5	20	9.5	90.25
24	14	9.93	14	25	−11	121
25	13	9.24	8.5	11	−2.5	6.25
26	14	9.43	14	15	−1	1
27	14	7.86	14	2	12	144
28	15	7.25	20.5	1	19.5	380.25
29	17	9.89	27	24	3	9
30	19	8.91	29.5	9	20.5	420.25
$\Sigma d_i^2 =$						**4016.5**

Given $T < Tc$ ($14.5 < 15, n = 15$), the difference of the *transverse diameter of the quadriceps belly* between *negatives and positives* was *statistically significant* at $< .01$.

The magnitude was:

$d = W / S = 91 / 120 =$ **0.76**.

– / +
negatives and positives

d
difference

| d |
absolute difference

n
sample size

R
relaxation
of the quadriceps mechanism

T
smaller sum of W– and W+ ranks

φ
transverse diameter
of the quadriceps belly
(cm)

W
sum of signed ranks of difference

n				φ	Ranks	Signed ranks	W−	W+
	***R*−**	***R*+**	***d***	$\lvert d \rvert$				
1	9.34	9.53	−0.19	0.19	5.5	−5.5	−5.5	2
2	8.21	8.05	0.16	0.16	2	2	−3.5	1
3	10.05	10.02	0.03	0.03	1	1	−5.5	8
4	9.96	9.72	0.24	0.24	8	8		13
5	10.06	9.25	0.81	0.81	13	13		10
6	9.84	9.3	0.54	0.54	10	10		9
7	8.99	8.6	0.39	0.39	9	9		15
8	9.46	8.39	1.07	1.07	15	15		3.5
9	9.48	9.66	−0.18	0.18	3.5	−3.5		11
10	8.18	8	0.18	0.18	3.5	3.5		7
11	10.33	9.73	0.6	0.6	11	11		12
12	9.93	9.7	0.23	0.23	7	7		14
13	9.24	9.43	−0.19	0.19	5.5	−5.5		
14	7.86	7.25	0.61	0.61	12	12		
15	9.89	8.91	0.98	0.98	14	14		
120						91	**−14.5**	105.5

Next internal confounder was the *patellar yaw* (PY) *according to Nove-Josserand and Dejour* (Nove-Josserand and Dejour, 1995).

The PY was an angle between the transverse axis of the patella on the CT image with the *greatest transverse diameter of the patella*, and the posterior intercondylar line connecting two most prominent points of the posterior parts of femoral condyles (Fig. 55).

Given that the patella was always inclined towards the *outer* side, that is to say *laterally*, the value of the angle was always *positive*.*

* There are several ways to measure the angle of patellar yaw. This is one of the oldest, and possibly one of the most utilized ways to do it in daily clinical practice, independent of FTD. Some ascribe this angle to the renowned Yale's professor of orthopedics and rehabilitation, John Pryor Fulkerson (1946–).

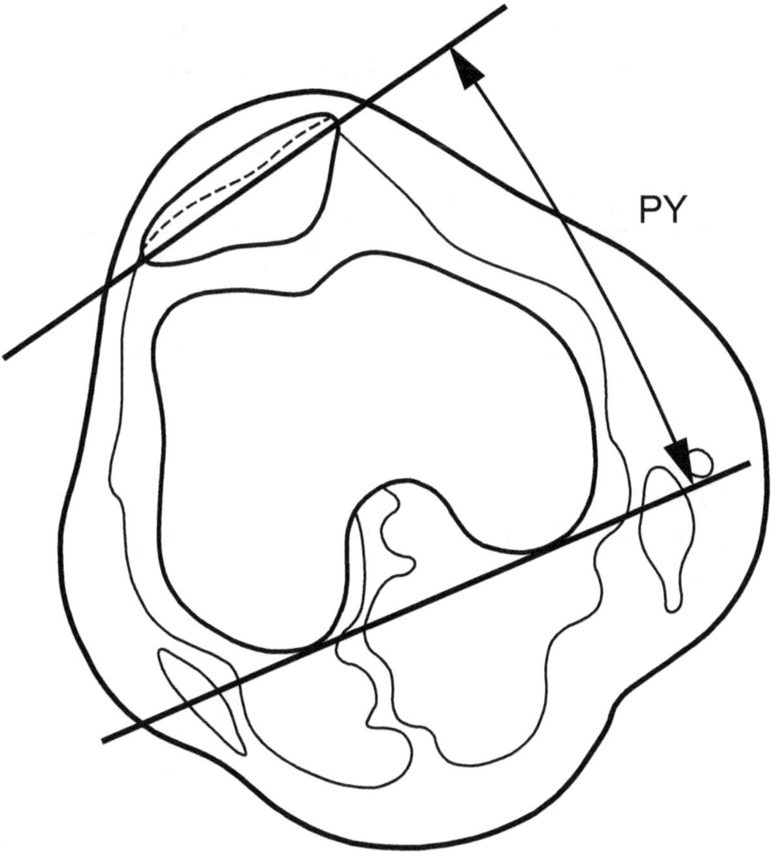

PY .... patellar yaw (according to Nove-Josserand and Dejour)

Fig. 55. Patellar yaw according to Nove-Josserand and Dejour

The Spearman's ρ for rank correlation between the *indicator* and the *patellar yaw according to Nove-Josserand and Dejour* was:

$$\rho = 1 - \frac{6 \times \sum d_i^2}{n \times (n^2 - 1)} = 1 - \frac{6 \times 3598.5}{30 \times (30^2 - 1)} = 1 - \frac{21591}{30 \times (900 - 1)}$$

$$= 1 - \frac{21591}{30 \times 899} = 1 - \frac{21591}{26970} = 1 - 0.80 = \mathbf{0.20}.$$

Given $\rho < \rho c$ (.20 < .47), the Spearman's correlation was not statistically significant at < .01. The magnitude was, also, 0.20.

d_i
rank difference

n
sample size (knees)

PY
patellar yaw
according to Nove-Josserand and Dejour in negatives and positives
(°)

TT–TIM
tibial tuberosity
–tibial intercondylar midpoint distance
in negatives and positives
(the indicator)
(mm)

n	Relaxation		Ranks		d_i	d_i^2
	TT-TIM	*PY*	*TT-TIM*	*PY*		
1	16	24.0	25	13	12	144
2	14	13.7	14	3	11	121
3	12	13.9	5.5	4	1.5	2.25
4	13	12.1	8.5	1	7.5	56.25
5	18	23.5	28	12	16	256
6	15	31.4	20.5	20	0.5	0.25
7	13	21.6	8.5	9	−0.5	0.25
8	14	22.9	14	10	4	16
9	11	36.2	3.5	24	−20.5	420.25
10	15	45.9	20.5	28	−7.5	56.25
11	14	29.3	14	15	−1	1
12	10	30.0	1.5	17.5	−16	256
13	15	40.7	20.5	26	−5.5	30.25
14	14	47.9	14	30	−16	256
15	11	23.4	3.5	11	−7.5	56.25
16	10	37.4	1.5	25	−23.5	552.25
17	16	30.0	25	17.5	7.5	56.25
18	15	20.6	20.5	8	12.5	156.25
19	15	34.0	20.5	23	−2.5	6.25
20	12	29.4	5.5	16	−10.5	110.25
21	16	13.3	25	2	23	529
22	13	16.2	8.5	5	3.5	12.25
23	19	31.5	29.5	21	8.5	72.25
24	14	25.5	14	14	0	0
25	13	16.3	8.5	6	2.5	6.25
26	14	19.0	14	7	7	49
27	14	45.5	14	27	−13	169
28	15	46.8	20.5	29	−8.5	72.25
29	17	33.0	27	22	5	25
30	19	30.5	29.5	19	10.5	110.25
$\Sigma d_i^2 =$						**3598.5**

Given $T > Tc$ ($40 > 15$, $n = 15$), the difference of the *patellar yaw according to Nove-Josserand and Dejour* between *negatives and positives* was *not statistically significant* at $< .01$.

The magnitude was:

$d = W / S = -36.7 / 120 = \mathbf{-0.31}$.

– / +
negatives and positives

d
difference

| d |
absolute difference

n
sample size

PY
patellar yaw
according to Nove-Josserand and Dejour
(°)

R
relaxation
of the quadriceps mechanism

T
smaller sum of W– and W+ ranks

W
sum of signed ranks of difference

n				PY	Ranks	Signed ranks	W−	W+
	R−	*R*+	*d*	|*d*|				
1	13.7	24	−10.3	10.3	14	−14	−14	4
2	13.9	12.1	1.8	1.8	4	4	−2.5	11
3	31.4	23.5	7.9	7.9	11	11	−13	1
4	21.6	22.9	−1.3	1.3	2.5	−2.5	−10	12
5	36.2	45.9	−9.7	9.7	13	−13	−15	7
6	30	29.3	0.7	0.7	1	1	−8	5
7	40.7	47.9	−7.2	7.2	10	−10	−9	
8	23.4	37.4	−14	14	15	−15	−6	
9	30	20.6	9.4	9.4	12	12	−2.5	
10	29.4	34	−4.6	4.6	8	−8		
11	16.2	13.3	2.9	2.9	7	7		
12	25.5	31.5	−6	6	9	−9		
13	16.3	19	−2.7	2.7	6	−6		
14	45.5	46.8	−1.3	1.3	2.5	−2.5		
15	33	30.5	2.5	2.5	5	5		
120						−36.7	−76.7	**40**

The *tendon yaw* (TY) *according to Šimunović* indicates the rotation of the inferior part of the quadriceps tendon in the transverse (axial) plane (Šimunović, 2023, p. 42).

The TY was an angle between the posterior intertendinous line connecting two most posterior points of the inferior part of the quadriceps tendon and the posterior intercondylar line of the proximal part of the tibia on the 'headless cut' (*see* p. 59) (Fig. 56).

Given that the inferior part of the quadriceps tendon was always inclined towards the *outer* side, that is to say *laterally*, the value of the angle was always *positive*.

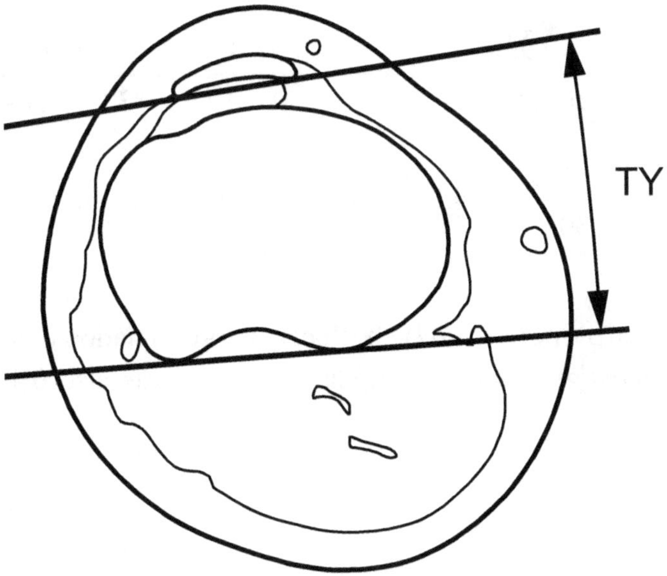

TY .... tendon yaw
(according to Šimunović)

Fig. 56. Tendon yaw according to Šimunović

The Spearman's ρ for rank correlation between the *indicator* and the *tendon yaw according to Šimunović* was:

$$\rho = 1 - \frac{6 \times \sum d_i^2}{n \times (n^2 - 1)} = 1 - \frac{6 \times 2328.5}{30 \times (30^2 - 1)} = 1 - \frac{13971}{30 \times (900 - 1)}$$

$$= 1 - \frac{13971}{30 \times 899} = 1 - \frac{13971}{26970} = 1 - 0.52 = \mathbf{0.48.}$$

Given $\rho > \rho c$ (.48 > .47), the Spearman's correlation was *statistically significant* at < .01. The magnitude was, also, 0.48.

d_i
rank difference

n
sample size (knees)

TT–TIM
tibial tuberosity
–tibial intercondylar midpoint distance
in negatives and positives
(the indicator)
(mm)

TY
tendon yaw
according to Šimunović
in negatives and positives
(°)

n	Relaxation		Ranks		d_i	d_i^2
	TT-TIM	*TY*	*TT-TIM*	*TY*		
1	16	12.7	25	9	16	256
2	14	13.7	14	11	3	9
3	12	15.5	5.5	16	−10.5	110.25
4	13	17.9	8.5	20	−11.5	132.25
5	18	21.8	28	25	3	9
6	15	20.2	20.5	23	−2.5	6.25
7	13	10.0	8.5	4	4.5	20.25
8	14	5.6	14	3	11	121
9	11	13.6	3.5	10	−6.5	42.25
10	15	21.2	20.5	24	−3.5	12.25
11	14	5.0	14	2	12	144
12	10	4.5	1.5	1	0.5	0.25
13	15	18.5	20.5	22	−1.5	2.25
14	14	27.0	14	30	−16	256
15	11	11.3	3.5	6	−2.5	6.25
16	10	14.3	1.5	13.5	−12	144
17	16	24.8	25	28	−3	9
18	15	23.1	20.5	27	−6.5	42.25
19	15	22.4	20.5	26	−5.5	30.25
20	12	18.0	5.5	21	−15.5	240.25
21	16	11.5	25	7	18	324
22	13	14.3	8.5	13.5	−5	25
23	19	26.4	29.5	29	0.5	0.25
24	14	14.9	14	15	−1	1
25	13	10.8	8.5	5	3.5	12.25
26	14	13.9	14	12	2	4
27	14	16.2	14	17.5	−3.5	12.25
28	15	11.8	20.5	8	12.5	156.25
29	17	16.2	27	17.5	9.5	90.25
30	19	17.4	29.5	19	10.5	110.25
$\Sigma d_i^2 =$						**2328.5**

Given T > Tc (36 > 15, n = 15), the difference of the *tendon yaw according to Šimunović* between *negatives and positives* was *not statistically significant* at < .01.

The magnitude was:

d = W / S = – 48 / 120 = **– 0.40**.

– / +
negatives and positives

d
difference

| d |
absolute difference

n
sample size

TY
tendon yaw
according to Šimunović
(°)

R
relaxation
of the quadriceps mechanism

T
smaller sum of W– and W+ ranks

W
sum of signed ranks of difference

n				**TY**	**Ranks**	**Signed ranks**	**W−**	**W+**
	R−	***R+***	***d***	**|*d*|**				
1	13.7	12.7	1	1	2	2	−6	2
2	15.5	17.9	−2.4	2.4	6	−6	−4	11
3	20.2	21.8	−1.6	1.6	4	−4	−13	5
4	10	5.6	4.4	4.4	11	11	−1	7
5	13.6	21.2	−7.6	7.6	13	−13	−14	11
6	4.5	5	−0.5	0.5	1	−1	−8	
7	18.5	27	−8.5	8.5	14	−14	−11	
8	11.3	14.3	−3	3	8	−8	−15	
9	24.8	23.1	1.7	1.7	5	5	−9	
10	18	22.4	−4.4	4.4	11	−11	−3	
11	14.3	11.5	2.8	2.8	7	7		
12	14.9	26.4	−11.5	11.5	15	−15		
13	10.8	13.9	−3.1	3.1	9	−9		
14	16.2	11.8	4.4	4.4	11	11		
15	16.2	17.4	−1.2	1.2	3	−3		
120						−48	−84	**36**

The *patellar riding* as an internal confounder to the indicator–condition relationship was evaluated according to the *Insall–Salvati* (IS) *ratio*, that is the ratio of the distance between the patellar base and the patellar apex as well as the distance between the patellar apex and the insertion of the inferior part of the quadriceps tendon (Insall and Salvati, 1971) (Fig. 57).*

The values **lower than 0.80** indicated a *low-riding patella*, that is to say: *patella infera* ('baja' /'baxa/, Spanish for 'low') whereas the values **greater than 1.20** indicated a *high-riding patella*, that is to say: *patella alta*. The ratio was, of course, *unitless*.

* There are several ways to assess patellar riding on XR and CT imaging. However, Insall-Salvatio ratio seems most reproducible of all adequate ratios. For more on this *see*, for example, Nizić *et al.*, 2014.

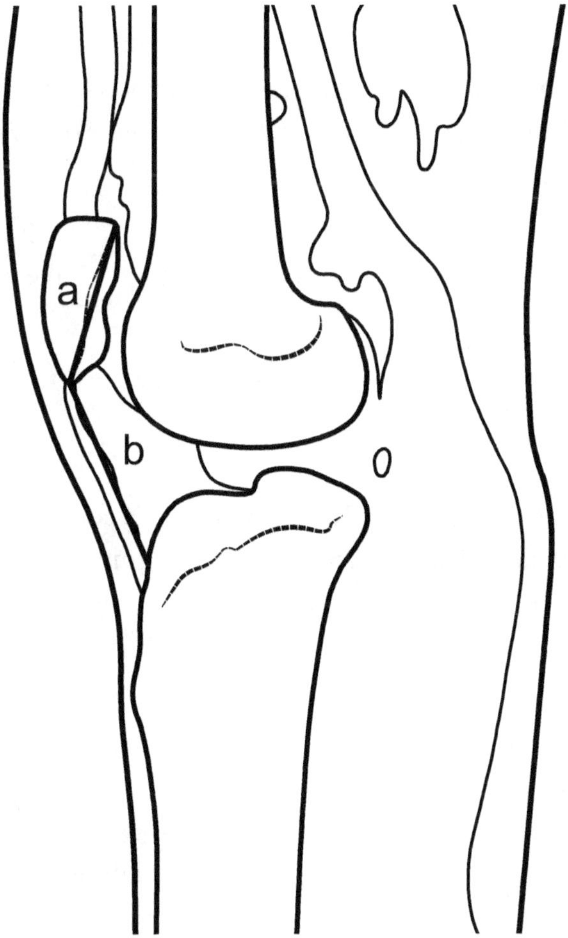

a........................the distance between the patellar base and the patellar apex
b............................ the distance between the patellar apex and the insertion of the inferior part of the quadriceps tendon

Fig. 57. Patellar riding according to Insall–Salvati ratio

The Spearman's ρ for rank correlation between the *indicator* and the *patellar riding according to Insall–Salvati ratio* was:

$$\rho = 1 - \frac{6 \times \sum d_i^2}{n \times (n^2 - 1)} = 1 - \frac{6 \times 3829.5}{30 \times (30^2 - 1)} = 1 - \frac{22977}{30 \times (900 - 1)}$$

$$= 1 - \frac{22977}{30 \times 899} = 1 - \frac{22977}{26970} = 1 - 0.85 = \mathbf{0.15}.$$

Given $\rho < \rho c$ (.15 < .47), the Spearman's correlation was *not statistically significant* at < .01. The magnitude was, also, 0.15.

d_i
rank difference

IS
patellar riding
according to Insal–Salvati ratio
in negatives and positives

n
sample size
(knees)

TT–TIM
tibial tuberosity
–tibial intercondylar midpoint distance
in negatives and positives
(the indicator)
(mm)

n	Relaxation		Ranks		d_i	d_i^2
	TT-TIM	*IS*	*TT-TIM*	*IS*		
1	16	0.986	25	8	17	289
2	14	0.996	14	9	5	25
3	12	0.923	5.5	4	1.5	2.25
4	13	0.985	8.5	7	1.5	2.25
5	18	1.032	28	13	15	225
6	15	1.132	20.5	21	−0.5	0.25
7	13	0.884	8.5	3	5.5	30.25
8	14	0.950	14	5	9	81
9	11	1.161	3.5	23	−19.5	380.25
10	15	1.259	20.5	28	−7.5	56.25
11	14	1.025	14	12	2	4
12	10	1.072	1.5	16	−14.5	210.25
13	15	1.119	20.5	19	1.5	2.25
14	14	1.076	14	17	−3	9
15	11	0.961	3.5	6	−2.5	6.25
16	10	1.057	1.5	15	−13.5	182.25
17	16	1.159	25	22	3	9
18	15	1.228	20.5	27	−6.5	42.25
19	15	1.120	20.5	20	0.5	0.25
20	12	1.051	5.5	14	−8.5	72.25
21	16	1.621	25	30	−5	25
22	13	1.181	8.5	26	−17.5	306.25
23	19	1.083	29.5	18	11.5	132.25
24	14	1.180	14	25	−11	121
25	13	1.002	8.5	10	−1.5	2.25
26	14	1.004	14	11	3	9
27	14	1.178	14	24	−10	100
28	15	1.382	20.5	29	−8.5	72.25
29	17	0.855	27	1	26	676
30	19	0.881	29.5	2	27.5	756.25
$\Sigma d_i^2 =$						**3829.5**

Given T > Tc (35 > 15, n = 15), the difference of the *patellar riding according to Insall–Salvati* between *negatives and positives* was *not statistically significant* at < .01.

The magnitude was:

d = W / S = – 50 / 120 = **– 0.42**.

– / +
negatives and positives

d
difference

| d |
absolute difference

IS
patellar riding
according to Insal–Salvati ratio

n
sample size
(participants)

R
relaxation
of the quadriceps mechanism

T
smaller sum of W– and W+ ranks

W
sum of signed ranks of difference

n				IS	Ranks	Signed ranks	W−	W+
	R−	*R*+	*d*	|*d*|				
1	0.996	0.986	0.010	0.010	2	2	−6	2
2	0.923	0.985	−0.062	0.062	6	−6	−7	13
3	1.132	1.032	0.100	0.100	13	13	−12	5
4	0.884	0.950	−0.066	0.066	7	−7	−10	4
5	1.161	1.259	−0.098	0.098	12	−12	−8.5	11
6	1.072	1.025	0.047	0.047	5	5	−8.5	
7	1.119	1.076	0.043	0.043	4	4	−15	
8	0.961	1.057	−0.096	0.096	10	−10	−1	
9	1.159	1.228	−0.069	0.069	8.5	−8.5	−14	
10	1.051	1.120	−0.069	0.069	8.5	−8.5	−3	
11	1.181	1.621	−0.440	0.440	15	−15		
12	1.18	1.083	0.097	0.097	11	11		
13	1.002	1.004	−0.002	0.002	1	−1		
14	1.178	1.382	−0.204	0.204	14	−14		
15	0.855	0.881	−0.026	0.026	3	−3		
120						−50	−85	**35**

The last internal confounder was the *tendon strain* (ε; Greek small letter 'epsilon'). The inferior part of the quadriceps tendon stretches during MVIC. In this small CT study, one wanted to see if this *stretching* had an important influence on the indicator–condition relationship.

The **strain** was contextualized as a linear deformation or, more precisely, longitudinal dilatation of a prismatic bar under axial weight-bearing conditions (Bazjanac, 1968, pp. 35, 47–8), calculated as follows:

$$\varepsilon = \frac{l_{\text{MVIC}} - l_{\text{R}}}{l_{\text{R}}} = \frac{\Delta l}{l_{\text{R}}}$$

where l_{MVIC} was the length of the inferior part of the quadriceps tendon during MVIC, and l_{R} was the length of the inferior part of the quadriceps tendon during relaxation of the quadriceps mechanism (Fig. 58a). The ratio was, of course, *unitless*.

The ε measurements were performed on 3D reconstructed CT images in the frontal plane.* The mean of the lentghs *a*, *b*, and *c* was the length of the inferior part of the tendon (Fig. 58b).

* In RadiAnt DICOM viewer (version 2022.1.1, 32-bit; 2009-2022 Medixant, Promienista 25, 60-288 Poznań, Poland), choose 3D volume rendering (F3) > 3D rotate (R) > Anterior (1) for each knee to get a unified measurement position, and then adjust manually for the tendon view.

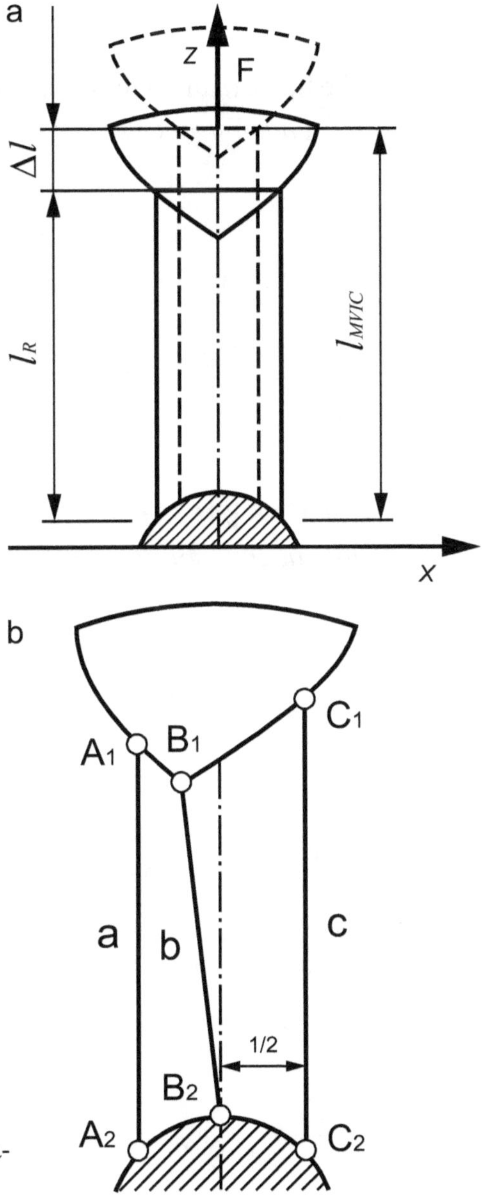

a, c .... lateral distances (margins)
b................. distance between the patellar apex (point B_1) and the middle of the inferior part of the quadriceps tendon on the tibial tuberosity (point B_2)
Δl .... difference between the l_R and l_{MVIC}
F .... force (direction of strain)
l_{MVIC} .... length of the inferior part of the quadriceps tendon during maximum voluntary isometric contraction of the quadriceps mechanism
l_R .... length of the inferior part of the quadriceps tendon during relaxation of the quadriceps mechanism
x-z .... axes (of the orthogonal coordinate system)

Fig. 58. The principle (**a**) and the measurement (**b**) of the tendon strain

The Spearman's ρ for rank correlation between the *indicator* and *tendon strain* was:

$$\rho = 1 - \frac{6 \times \sum d_i^2}{n \times (n^2 - 1)} = 1 - \frac{6 \times 2933.5}{30 \times (30^2 - 1)} = 1 - \frac{17601}{30 \times (900 - 1)}$$

$$= 1 - \frac{17601}{30 \times 899} = 1 - \frac{17601}{26970} = 1 - 0.65 = \mathbf{0.35}.$$

Given $\rho < \rho c$ (.35 < .47), the Spearman's correlation was *not statistically significant* at < .01. The magnitude was, also, 0.35.

d_i
rank difference

ε
tendon strain
in negatives and positives

n
sample size
(knees)

TT–TIM
tibial tuberosity
–tibial intercondylar midpoint distance
in negatives and positives
(the indicator)
(mm)

n	Relaxation		Ranks		d_i	d_i^2
	TT-TIM	ε	*TT-TIM*	ε		
1	16	0.20	25	20.5	4.5	20.25
2	14	0.10	14	7	7	49
3	12	0.02	5.5	2.5	3	9
4	13	0.03	8.5	4.5	4	16
5	18	0.36	28	30	−2	4
6	15	0.23	20.5	22	−1.5	2.25
7	13	0.19	8.5	18.5	−10	100
8	14	0.24	14	23	−9	81
9	11	0.13	3.5	11.5	−8	64
10	15	0.16	20.5	16.5	4	16
11	14	0.12	14	9	5	25
12	10	0.20	1.5	20.5	−19	361
13	15	0.12	20.5	9	11.5	132.25
14	14	0.12	14	9	5	25
15	11	0.28	3.5	26	−22.5	506.25
16	10	0.02	1.5	2.5	−1	1
17	16	0.30	25	27.5	−2.5	6.25
18	15	0.26	20.5	24.5	−4	16
19	15	0.33	20.5	29	−8.5	72.25
20	12	0.30	5.5	27.5	−22	484
21	16	0.14	25	14	11	121
22	13	0.14	8.5	14	−5.5	30.25
23	19	0.16	29.5	16.5	13	169
24	14	0.13	14	11.5	2.5	6.25
25	13	0.14	8.5	14	−5.5	30.25
26	14	0.06	14	6	8	64
27	14	0.01	14	1	13	169
28	15	0.03	20.5	4.5	16	256
29	17	0.19	27	18.5	8.5	72.25
30	19	0.26	29.5	24.5	5	25
$\Sigma d_i^2 =$						**2933.5**

Given T > Tc (38 > 9, n = 13), the difference of the *tendon strain* between *negatives and positives* was *not statistically significant* at < .01.

The magnitude was:

d = W / S = – 15 / 102 = **– 0.15**.

– / +
negatives and positives

†
excluded (zero) ranks

d
difference

| d |
absolute difference

ε
tendon strain

n
sample size
(participants)

T
smaller sum of W– and W+ ranks

W
sum of signed ranks of difference

n				ε	Ranks	Signed ranks	W−	W+
	−	+	*d*	|*d*|				
1	0.10	0.20	−0.10	0.10	11	−11	−11	9.5
2	0.02	0.03	−0.01	0.01	1	−1	−1	13
3	0.23	0.36	−0.13	0.13	12	−12	−12	6
4	0.19	0.24	−0.05	0.05	7	−7	−7	9.5
5	0.13	0.16	−0.03	0.03	4	−4	−4	
6	0.20	0.12	0.08	0.08	9.5	9.5	−4	
7 †	0.12	0.12	0	0	—	—	−4	
8	0.28	0.02	0.26	0.26	13	13	−2	
9	0.30	0.26	0.04	0.04	6	6	−8	
10	0.30	0.33	−0.03	0.03	4	−4		
11 †	0.14	0.14	0	0	—	—		
12	0.13	0.16	−0.03	0.03	4	−4		
13	0.14	0.06	0.08	0.08	9.5	9.5		
14	0.01	0.03	−0.02	0.02	2	−2		
15	0.19	0.26	−0.07	0.07	8	−8		
102						−15	−53	**38**

It is, therefore, notable that transverse diameter of the quadriceps belly, hence the quadriceps strength, had a bioimportant effect on the condition whereas **none** of the internal confounders had a large influence on the indicator, the TT-TIM distance. This is especially true if one takes into account all magnitudes **would shrink in larger samples**, thus making the effect even less important than shown in Fig. 59.*

* In his thesis, Šimunović found the transverse area of the *vastus medialis obliquus* muscle did not influence lateral patellar tilt. In this small CT study, on the contrary, the transverse diameter of the quadriceps belly has emerged as the most important influence on the condition. However, the measurement comprised *all* four heads of the muscle at yet another measurement level. It might be reasonable to speculate the vastus medialis obliquus *alone* does not influence the patellar yaw; the interplay of all quadriceps heads might be responsible for this impact, perhaps mostly the interchange between the vastus lateralis and vastus medialis obliquus. It is an open question of cause and effect: does the weak quadriceps cause the condition or the condition, caused, for example, by FTD, propagates sparing of the knee and thus hypotrophy of the quadriceps mechanism, only to further aggravate the condition? If hypotrophy came first, as FTDs are frequent, yet mild, the question is what caused the strongest muscle in the human body to become weak to begin with? If FTD came first, causing repetitive patellar dislocations, so the patient did not use the leg as often and hypotrophy of the quadriceps ensued, the question is what caused FTD to begin with? The average patients's age is telling. We know symmetry is Nature's signature in biosystems. The quadriceps muscles should develop symmetrically on each side, and their transverse diameters should be equal at the same measurement level, yet variations are imminent, perhaps too great and not so apparent at first. With development and growth, they become more debilitating as growing in height *decreases* the already insufficient transverse diameter and causes quadriceps on one side to lag behind, to become weaker, deepening the femoral trochlea with lesser strength, hence FTD (unilateral FTD in knee pairs proves this). Most FTDs are mild, presenting with a groove not enough scooped out. It might be the weak muscle is the originator due to Nature's imperfect symmetric tendencies, as with brains, faces and breasts.

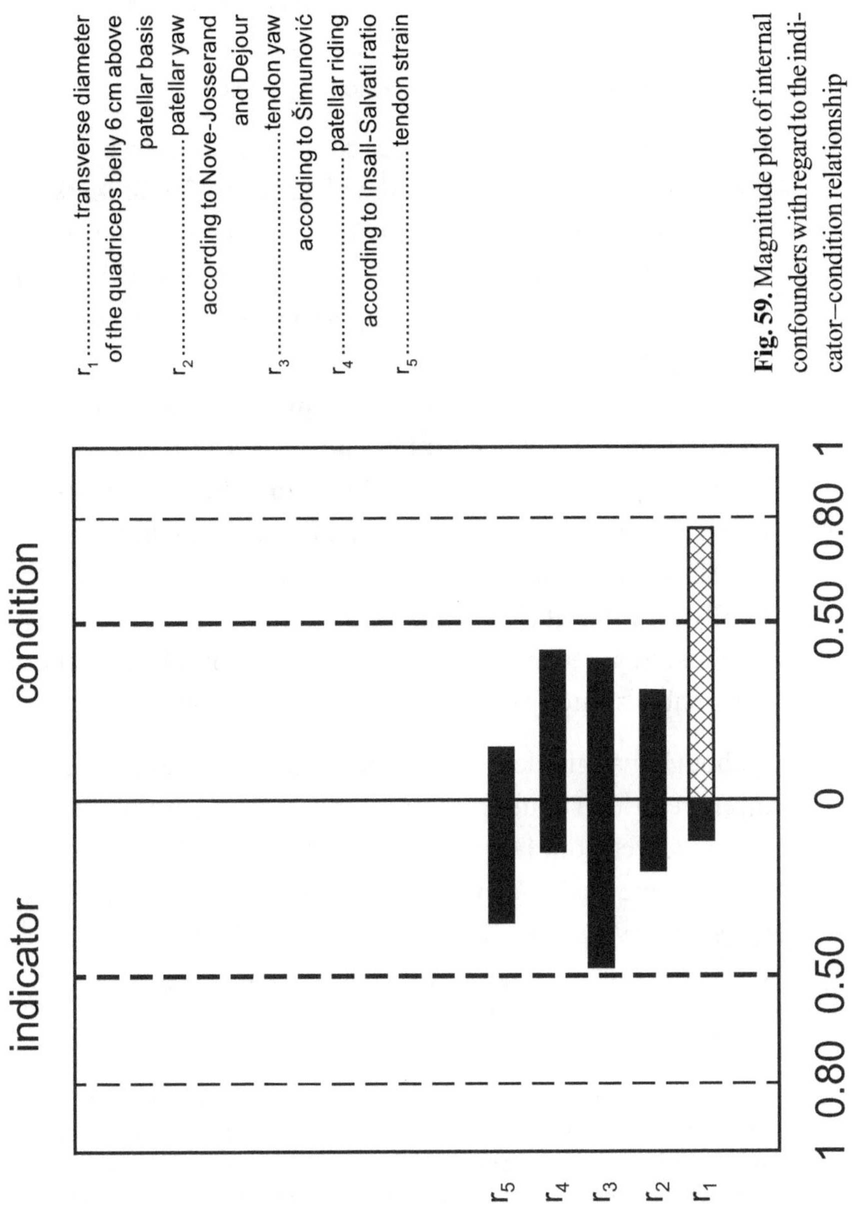

Fig. 59. Magnitude plot of internal confounders with regard to the indicator–condition relationship

Should one collect all confounders to the indicator and the condition in this small CT study to show them in a single magnitude plot, it would look like the one in Fig. 60.

It is clear from the plot only three confounders deserve a more detailed investigation, marked with an asterisk (*): *sex* with regard to the indicator, and *transverse diameter of the quadriceps belly* as well as *FTD* with regard to the condition. All the other ties are *theoretically* important, especially considering larger sample size would further *decrease* their magnitudes. **This simply means indicator needs a *sex-split cut-off* whereas the condition might be caused by the *hypotrophy of the entire quadriceps belly* and, to a somewhat lesser extent, *FTD*.** Taking into account most FTDs are *mild*, however, it appears **quadriceps belly weakness could be the most practically important effect** causing the condition which, in turn, implies strengthening the entire quadriceps muscle might be a reasonable strategy in conservative therapeutic approach.

Although magnitudes will *decrease* with larger samples, their interpretation should remain *equal*, and no amount of further research could negate these findings. In other words: if the same methodology were to be followed in larger samples, the *interpretation* of magnitudes (and not their exact values!) should be similar, if not identical.* Statistical significance is, nevertheless, of secondary import.

* Using different methodology would give different results. This is, I gather, self-explanatory, though it sometimes amazes me how this logical rule is overlooked. Should one desire to replicate the findings of this small CT study, it should be done following the *same* methodology, and in no other way!

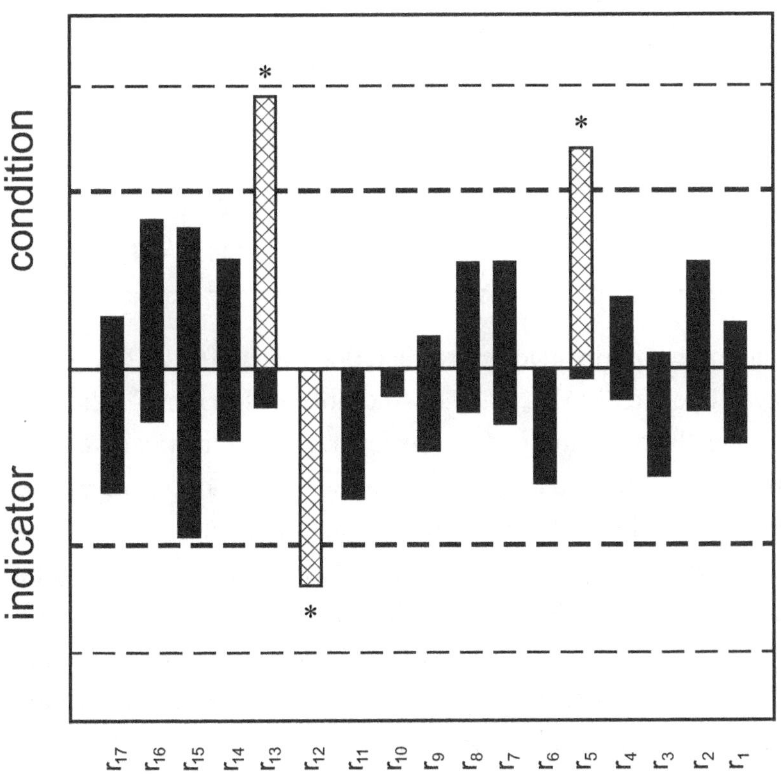

r_1 .... femoral rotation (angle)
r_2 .... tibial rotation (angle)
r_3 .... knee rotation (angle)
r_4 .... tibial torsion (angle) (at the level of the tibial tuberosity)
r_5 .... sulcus angle (femoral trochlear dysplasia)
r_6 .... extension angle (flexion–extension of the knee)
r_7 .... joint line convergence angle (varus–valgus deformity)
r_8 .... medial plateau posterior tibial slope (angle)
r_9 .... lateral plateau posterior tibial slope (angle)
r_{10} .... age
r_{11} .... body side
r_{12} .... sex
r_{13} .... transverse diameter of the quadriceps belly 6 cm above the patellar basis
r_{14} .... patellar yaw according to Nove-Josserand and Dejour
r_{15} .... tendon yaw according to Šimunović
r_{16} .... patellar riding according to Insall-Salvati ratio
r_{17} .... tendon strain

Fig. 60. Magnitude plot of external and internal confounders with regard to the indicator–condition relationship

n				φ	Ranks	Signed ranks	W−	W+
	R−	*R*+	*d*	|*d*|				
1	9.34	9.53	−0.19	0.19	5.5	−5.5	−5.5	2
2	8.21	8.05	0.16	0.16	2	2	−3.5	1
3	10.05	10.02	0.03	0.03	1	1	−5.5	8
4	9.96	9.72	0.24	0.24	8	8		13
5	10.06	9.25	0.81	0.81	13	13		10
6	9.84	9.30	0.54	0.54	10	10		9
7	8.99	8.60	0.39	0.39	9	9		15
8	9.46	8.39	1.07	1.07	15	15		3.5
9	9.48	9.66	−0.18	0.18	3.5	−3.5		11
10	8.18	8.00	0.18	0.18	3.5	3.5		7
11	10.33	9.73	0.6	0.6	11	11		12
12	9.93	9.70	0.23	0.23	7	7		14
13	9.24	9.43	−0.19	0.19	5.5	−5.5		
14	7.86	7.25	0.61	0.61	12	12		
15	9.89	8.91	0.98	0.98	14	14		
120						91	**−14.5**	105.5

The magnitude of φ in quadriceps relaxation was 0.76 (p. 202) whereas its magnitude after MVIC was 0.62 (the table on the right). Therefore, on average, the magnitude of φ between negatives and positives was **0.69** ((0.76+0.62)/2). This magnitude was, without a doubt, a *large* one. However, this effect was due to measuring the diameter of the muscle belly. **During clinical examination, an orthopedic surgeon can evaluate only the leg, and not the muscle diameter.** How does, then, the state of affairs look like if one would to measure the diameter of the *entire leg at the same measurement level* used to measure the diameter of the quadriceps muscle belly?

n				φ	Ranks	Signed ranks	W−	W+
	MVIC−	*MVIC+*	*d*	*|d|*				
1	8.2	8.1	0.1	0.1	1	1	−11	1
2	8.2	8.0	0.2	0.2	3	3	−12	3
3	10.6	10.3	0.3	0.3	6	6		6
4	9.4	9.2	0.2	0.2	3	3		3
5	9.4	8.7	0.7	0.7	9.5	9.5		9.5
6	9.2	8.5	0.7	0.7	9.5	9.5		9.5
7	8.6	8.1	0.5	0.5	8	8		8
8	8.7	8.4	0.3	0.3	6	6		6
9	8.9	8.7	0.2	0.2	3	3		3
10	7.8	7.5	0.3	0.3	6	6		6
11	9.8	7.5	2.3	2.3	15	15		15
12	10.4	9.0	1.4	1.4	13	13		13
13	8.8	9.6	−0.8	0.8	11	−11		14
14	7.7	8.6	−0.9	0.9	12	−12		
15	8.8	7.1	1.7	1.7	14	14		
120						74	**−23**	97

Given T > Tc (23 > 15, n = 15), the difference of the *transverse diameter of the quadriceps belly* between *negatives and positives after MVIC* was *not statistically significant* at < .01.

The magnitude was:

d = W / S = 74 / 120 = **0.62**.

In the transverse plane, on the '6-cut' CT image, the horizontal distance between two vertical diagonals was the *transverse diameter of the leg* (Φ; Greek capital letter 'phi') in *centimeters*. In this small CT study, in all thirty knees, it was a rather quick and easy measurement (Fig. 61).

Hence, upon MVIC, one expects the value of Φ to *decrease*.

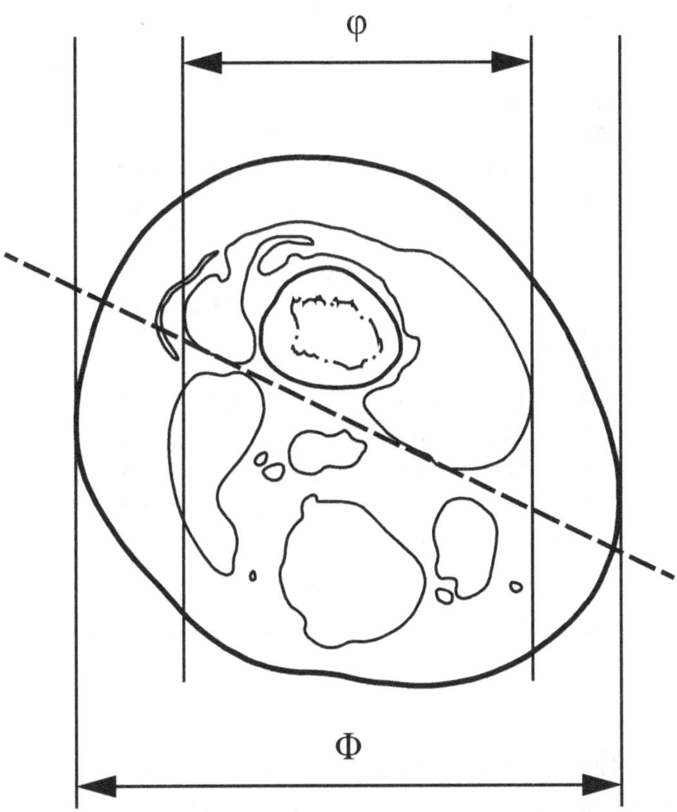

φ ....transverse diameter of the quadriceps belly

Φ........................transverse diameter of the leg

Fig. 61. Measurement of the transverse diameter of the quadriceps belly and the leg on the '6-cut' transverse CT image

n				Φ	Ranks	Signed ranks	W−	W+
	R−	*R*+	*d*	|*d*|				
1	12.7	13.0	−0.3	0.3	8.5	−8.5	−8.5	3.5
2	10.5	10.4	0.1	0.1	3.5	3.5	−8.5	3.5
3	15.8	15.7	0.1	0.1	3.5	3.5	−3.5	15
4	13	13.3	−0.3	0.3	8.5	−8.5	−3.5	11.5
5	11.6	10.9	0.7	0.7	15	15		8.5
6	12	11.6	0.4	0.4	11.5	11.5		13
7	11.7	11.4	0.3	0.3	8.5	8.5		3.5
8	14	13.5	0.5	0.5	13	13		3.5
9	13.2	13.1	0.1	0.1	3.5	3.5		14
10	11.1	11.0	0.1	0.1	3.5	3.5		8.5
11	13.5	13.6	−0.1	0.1	3.5	−3.5		11.5
12	13.7	13.1	0.6	0.6	14	14		
13	12.3	12.4	−0.1	0.1	3.5	−3.5		
14	11.5	11.2	0.3	0.3	8.5	8.5		
15	12	11.6	0.4	0.4	11.5	11.5		
120						72	**−24**	96

Given T > Tc (24 > 15, n = 15), the difference of the *transverse diameter of the leg* between *negatives and positives in quadriceps relaxation* was *not statistically significant* at < .01.

The magnitude was:

d = W / S = 72 / 120 = **0.60**.

n	*MVIC–*	*MVIC+*	*d*	**Φ** $\lvert d \rvert$	**Ranks**	**Signed ranks**	**W–**	**W+**
1	12.2	12.6	−0.4	0.4	9	−9	−9	1.5
2	10.5	10.4	0.1	0.1	1.5	1.5	−13	14.5
3	16.3	16.9	−0.6	0.6	13	−13	−5.5	9
4	12	12.3	−0.3	0.3	5.5	−5.5	−5.5	9
5	11.3	10.5	0.8	0.8	14.5	14.5		11.5
6	11.6	11.2	0.4	0.4	9	9		5.5
7	11.4	11	0.4	0.4	9	9		3
8	13.9	13.4	0.5	0.5	11.5	11.5		14.5
9	12.8	12.5	0.3	0.3	5.5	5.5		1.5
10	10.8	10.6	0.2	0.2	3	3		5.5
11	13.5	13.8	−0.3	0.3	5.5	−5.5		11.5
12	13.8	13	0.8	0.8	14.5	14.5		
13	12.5	12.4	0.1	0.1	1.5	1.5		
14	11.3	11	0.3	0.3	5.5	5.5		
15	11.4	10.9	0.5	0.5	11.5	11.5		
120						54	**−33**	87

Given T > Tc (33 > 15, n = 15), the difference of the *transverse diameter of the leg* between *negatives and positives after MVIC* was *not statistically significant* at < .01.

The magnitude was:

d = W / S = 54 / 120 = **0.45**.

Therefore, on average, one could clearly see the effect of measuring the diameter of the quadriceps muscle belly (.69) was *greater* than that of the entire leg (.53; (0.60+0.45)/2). The average difference was .16, still the magnitude increased for 30% (0.69–0.53=0.16; 0.16/0.53 = 0.30 × 100% = 30%). Given that 33% is one third of the cases, a **30% increase** would be reasonably labeled as **substantial**. This would imply the recognition of quadriceps belly hypotrophy would be about 30% easier if the diameter of the quadriceps muscle belly were measured. Using visual evaluation during clinical examination, especially if quadriceps muscles are contracted, might not be sensitive enough to recognize hypotrophy of the quadriceps belly. This, in turn implies **quadriceps hypotrophy is much more frequent, yet *subclinical* and, thus, *underreported*.**

If one were to look at the data, those in quadriceps relaxation, for example, 73% (11/15) of positives did, and 27% (4/15) did not have leg hypotrophy of different scale. However, only 36% (4/11) of those 73% were reported in orthopedic charts (Fig. 62). **In conclusion, this implies clinical evaluation is not sensitive enough, underestimating the *prevalence* of leg hypotrophy, and hence the hypotrophy of the entire quadriceps muscle belly as the largest effect tied with recurrent patellar dislocation.**

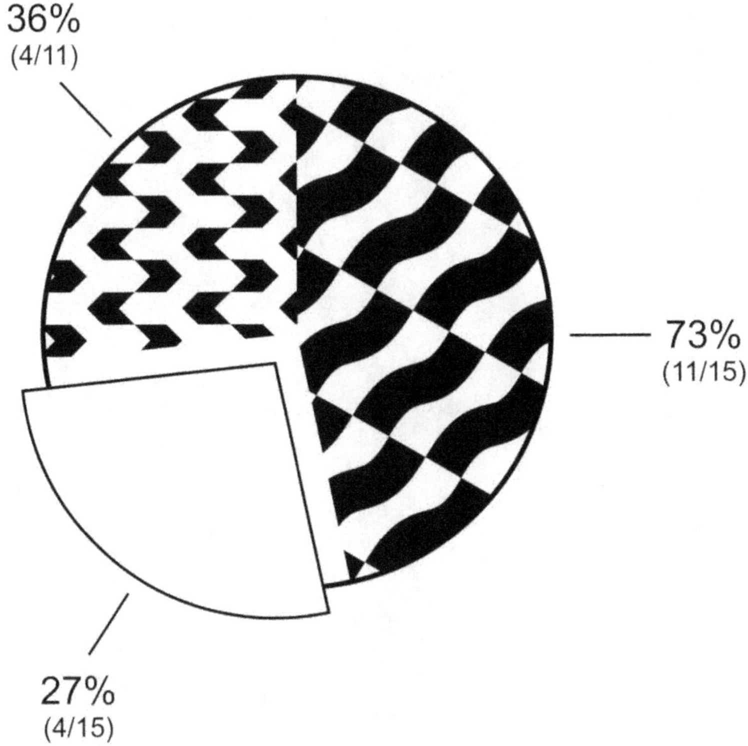

Fig. 62. Pie chart of sample knees with leg hypotrophy in quadriceps muscle relaxation

4

Commentary

According to what magnitudes were able to demonstrate as well as suggest, the most probable cause of the condition (recurrent patellar dislocation) would be a hypotrophy of the quadriceps muscle belly that is often **subclinical**, and thus not recognized in clinical examination. At first presentation, the average patient is a female adolescent. A unilateral diameter of the quadriceps muscle belly was probably smaller beforehand due to Nature's tendency for imperfect (variable) symmetry, hence the muscle on one side of the body was weaker. Growing in height is nothing more than a longitudinal dilatation of a prismatic bar (the quadriceps muscle belly) under axial weight-bearing conditions that is known to simultanously cause transverse contraction, in other words **decrease** of the transverse diameter of the quadriceps muscle belly, hence further causing its weakness.* The patella, a part of the quadriceps muscle, could be regarded as a *grooving plane*. Years of daily activities preceding presentation (such as walking, running, and so on) made the weaker muscle less capable to plane the groove of the femoral trochlea, so it became shallower than it would otherwise be. This shallowness, coupled with muscular weakness caused the first patellar dislocation, starting

* The longitudinal dilatation and transverse contraction form a ratio depending on the type of the material, *m* or *Poisson's number*, with 1 / m being the *Poisson's coefficient,* after Siméon Denis Poisson (1781–1840), French physicist and mathematician (for most materials, *m* = 3 : 4). For more on this, *see* Bazjanac, 1968, p. 36.

a 'vicious circle': the patient was sparing the painful knee, the quadriceps muscle belly got weaker causing another patellar dislocation with patient sparing the knee even more only to make the muscle weaker for another patellar dislocation to occur, and so on.

Logically, the first thing to do would be to **recognize** the patient, and then **strengthen** the quadriceps muscle (certainly not to deepen the trochlear groove of the femur because most of the patients' grooves are just a bit shallow, with no major irregularities). To adequatelly manage the patient, the imaging indicator must recognize the patient and inform the clinican whether or not the patient is doing better after therapy. In practice, this would mean the value of the indicator should **decrease** after therapy in the same imaging conditions if the strengthening of the quadriceps muscle belly were successful. Therefore, the **simple clinical algorithm** could look like this:

1) Measure the indicator (TT-TIM distance, for example). If pathological, exercise strenghtening of the quadriceps muscle belly for *three months*.

2) After three months, measure the indicator again. If the value of the indicator *decreased* enough to become physiological, the patient is cured.

3) If the value of the indicator decreased, but not enough to become physiological, *repeat* the procedure!

The standard indicator (TT-TG distance) cannot be used in such a manner. **TT-TG distance is an indicator of FTD, and not the condition (recurrent patellar dislocation).** Only because FTD mostly goes **in tandem** with the condition, TT-TG distance is able to **indirectly** recognize the condition. However, since its TG point is not static, it cannot recognize if the insertion of the quadriceps mechanism (the TT point) has changed its location.** This implies it could not control the therapeutic outcome conservative or surgical alike because both change the location of the insertion—they both **medialize** it. In this small CT study, the indicator, the TT-TIM distance, had an (overall) **accuracy >70%** (74%), the highest **precision** among similar indicators (sd = 2.8 mm) and detected the change of insertional location. When sex-split cut offs were used (**15 mm** for **males** and **12 mm** for **females**), **sensitivity** was **around 60%** (60% and 62%, respectively) and **specificity** was **around 80%** (80% and 76%, respectively). The results seem promising and demonstrate the sorting and tracking validity of the TT-TIM distance in daily clinical practice. Of course, further research should be undertaken to elucidate important aspects uncovered in this small CT study.

** The fact that TT-TG distance is not reactive to the quadriceps contraction was erroneously perceived as advantageous because no additional CT scanning during MVIC should have been required. This notion illustrates how interpretation is, by far, the main chalenge of scientific research.

The fact TT-TIM distance *recognized the positives* (d = –.80), as well as *decreased after MVIC* (d = 0.71) (as it logically should have) means it may have enough sorting and tracking validity in clinical practice to represent a possible benchmark in gauging a therapeutic outcome, especially that of conservative nature which might be a preferred type of patient management to begin with.

TT-TIM distance seems as *accurate* as TT-TG distance, only more specific, way more *precise*, practically *independent* of the plethora of many different confounders and can be *reliably* measured on the Siemens 16-row CT scanner.

5

5

Afterword

Afterword

The scientific field of patellofemoral research is complicated. New papers are published every day, and, for the most part, it boils down to statistical testing of various relationships of interest. Fifteen years ago, when I got into the field, one could rather easily grasp the most essential scientific work on the topic. Today, however, the body of literature has grown so vast it is becoming increasingly difficult to keep pace. Yet, in the midst of all the new scientific production, nothing of essence has changed. At times, the field may appear as a giant conundrum where one fails to understand what is practically important. And that is exactly why a researcher should investigate—to find a *practically important effect.*

A *magnitude* is the size of an effect, the so called *effect size*, be it a correlation or a difference. It is a word most often related to *earthquakes*. In this small CT study, I used magnitudes to understand which relationships of interest regarding the indicator (the TT-TIM distance) and the condition (the recurrent patellar dislocations) are more practically important than others.

The idea magnitudes could help with clearing things up came from the actual earthquake I witnessed in Zagreb, on Sunday, the 22nd of March 2020. Looking at the cracked walls of my apartment made me realize that the higher magnitude might have been fatal. And *voilà*—the *magnitude*!

An even stranger event brought an idea of an *invisible wall.* One afternoon I was drinking coffee with a friend of mine in my neighborhood's coffee-shop. The weather was wonderful, and we were sitting outside. Behind my back, there was a transparent Perspex wall. Suddenly, I felt a strong blow. A crow crashed into the wall and broke her neck. This bizarre incident got me thinking one could die from hitting a wall one cannot see. And *voilà*—an *invisible wall* (the *ball* was just a rhyme away!). This goes to say seemingly unconnected events may be a fertile soil for new paradigms. Newton had his apple, Einstein had his trains whereas all I had was an earthquake and a dead crow.

I have begun researching patellofemoral instability in 2010. It was an anecdotal start—the most powerful authority figure of the musculoskeletal radiology in the country at the time graced me with 'Her Majesty's' approval allowing me to investigate it because, quite frankly, nobody was eager to do it. It was far too entangled! I had no resources whatsoever, yet gathered a decent number of hurdles along the way. Not to mention I had not had the faintest idea how to do research! I have trained myself in biostatistics as well as foreign academic writing on the fly, reading long hours in my spare time. Nevertheless, nothing would give me more pleasure other than fellow researchers investigating TT-TIM distance to a much greater extent around the world, with an honest understanding it may appear to have a serious potential in resolving the patellofemoral diagnostic puzzle. I hope this small CT study would become a helpful step along the way.

This booklet, as well as much of the pertinent work in the past would not see the light of day without the constant help of my friend and colleague radiologist, Marko Šimunović, MD, PhD, and likewise my mentor, orthopedic surgeon professor Mislav Jelić, MD, PhD. I hereby thank the reviewers for making this booklet a smoother read.

Lastly, I am especially thankful to the surgical reviewer, Mario Josipović, MD, PhD, an excellent orthopedic surgeon, for writing a thoughtful foreword.

The Author

In *Zagreb*, September 2025

6

6

Bibliography

books & papers

Bibliography

Al-Alwan HAS, Al-Bazzaz IA, Ali YHM. The potency of architectural probabilism in shaping cognitive environments: a psychophysical approach. *Ain Shams Engineering Journal*. 2022;13(1):1–11. DOI: 10.1016/j.asej.2021.06.008.

Altman DG. Practical statistics for medical research. Boca Raton, FL: *Chapman & Hall/CRC*. 1999. DOI: 10.1201/9780429258589.

Andrejev V. Mehanika. II. dio. Kinematika. Zagreb: *Tehnička knjiga*. 1971.

Bae K, Aldosari AM, Kang MS. The difference in tibial tuberosity to trochlear groove distance between CT and MRI arises from the degree of knee flexion during imaging. *J Pediatr Orthop*. 2023;43(9):e761–8. DOI: 10.1097/BPO.0000000000002481.

Bazjanac D. Nauka o čvrstoći. Zagreb: *Tehnička knjiga*. 1968.

Bazjanac D. Tehnička mehanika. I. dio. Statika. Zagreb: *Tehnička knjiga*. 1966.

Bazjanac D. Tehnička mehanika. II dio. Kinematika. Zagreb: *Tehnička knjiga*. 1977.

Benjamin DJ, Berger JO, Johannesson M, Nosek BA, Wagenmakers EJ, Berk R, Bollen Ka, Brembs B, Brown L, Camerer C, Cesarini D, Chambers CD, Clyde M, Cook TD, De Boeck P, Dienes Z, Dreber A, Easwaran K, Efferson C, Fehr E, Fidler F, Field AP, Foster M, George EI, Gonzalez R, Goodman S, Green E, Green DP, Greenwald AG, Hadfield JD, Hedges LV, Held L, Hua Ho T, Hoijtink H, Hrusch DJ, Imai K, Imbens G, Ioannidis JPA, Jeon M,

Jones JH, Kirchler M, Laibson D, List J, Little R, Lupia A, Machery E, Maxwell SE, McCarthy M, Moore DA, Morgan SL, Munafó M, Nakagawa S, Nyhan B, Parker TH, Pericchi L, Perugini M, Rouder J, Rousseau J, Savalei V, Schönbrodt FD, Sellke T, Sinclair B, Tingley D, Van Zandt T, Vazire S, Watts DJ, Winship C, Wolpert RL, Xie Y, Young C, Zinman J, Johnson VE. Redefine statistical significance. *Nat Hum Behav*. 2018;2(1):6–10. DOI: 10.1038/s41562-017-0189-z.

Bertoldo G, Zandonella Callegher C, Altoè G. Designing studies and evaluating research results: type M and type S error for Pearson correlation coefficient. *Meta-Psychology*. 2022; 6:MP.2020.2573:1–18. DOI: 10.15626/MP.2020.2573.

Biedert RM (ed). Patellofemoral disorders. Diagnosis and treatment. 1st ed. Chichester, UK: *John Wiley & Sons Ltd*. 2004. DOI: 10.1002/0470011165.

Binder D, Piecha T, Schroeder-Heister P (eds). The logical writings of Karl Popper. Trends in Logic. Studia Logica Library. Volume 58. Cham, SW: *Springer Nature Switzerland AG*. 2022. DOI: 10.1007/978-3-030-94926-6.

Camathias C, Pagenstert G, Stutz U, Barg A, Müller-Gerbl M, Nowakowski AM. The effect of knee flexion and rotation on the tibial tuberosity–trochlear groove distance. *Knee Surg Sports Traumatol Arthrosc*. 2016;24(9):2811–17. DOI: 10.1007/s00167-015-3508-9.

Canna SW, Chauvin NA, Burnham JM. A 17 year old with isolated proximal tibiofibular joint arthritis. *Pediatr Rheumatol*. 2013;11(1):1. DOI: 10.1186/1546-0096-11-1.

Carlson VR, Sheehan FT, Shen A, Yao L, Jackson JN, Boden BP. The relationship of static tibial tubercle–trochlear groove measurement and dynamic patellar tracking. *Am J Sports Med*. 2017;45(8):1856–63. DOI: 10.1177/0363546517700119.

Cline G. Nonparametric statistical methods using R. Waltham Abbey Essex, UK: *ED-Tech Press*, 2019.

Cohen J. Statistical power analysis for the behavioral sciences. 2nd ed. New York: *Lawrence Erlbaum Associates*. 1988. DOI: 10.4324/9780203771587.

Cusco X, Seijas R, Ares O, Cugat JR, Garcia-Balletbo M, Cugat R. Superior dislocation of the patella: a case report. *J Orthop Surg Res*. 2009;4:29. DOI: 10.1186/1749-799X-4-29.

Čaušević M. Tehnička mehanika. Kinematika. Zagreb: *Školska knjiga*. 2000.

Dahhan P, Delepine G, Larde D. L'articulation fémoro-patellaire. *Anat Clin*. 1981:3:23–38. DOI: 10.1007/BF01557971.

Dejour H, Carret JP, Walch G. Les 6èmes journées Lyonnaises de chirurgie du genou. Lyon: *Clinique de chirurgie orthopédique et traumatologique centre hospitalier Lyon–Sud*. 1987.

Fischer HR. Abductive reasoning as a way of worldmaking. *Foundations of Science*. 2001;6:361–83. DOI: 10.1023/A:1011671106610.

Gelman A, Carlin J. Beyond power calculations: assessing type S (sign) and type M (magnitude) errors. *Perspect Pscyhol Sci*. 2014;9(6):641–51. DOI: 10.1177/1745691614551642.

Glantz SA. Primer of biostatistics. 6th ed. New York: *McGraw-Hill*. 2005.

Gorski O, Majnarić N. Grčko-hrvatski rječnik. 8. izd. Zagreb: *Školska knjiga*. 2005.

Goutallier D, Bernageau J, Lecudonnec B. Mesure de l'écart tubérosité antérieure—gorge de la trochlée (T.A.-G.T.). Technique. Résultats. Intérêt. *Rev de Chirurgie Orthopedique*. 1978;64:423–8.

Greene WB, Heckman JD (eds). The clinical measurement of joint motion. Rosemont, IL: *American Academy of Orthopaedic Surgeons*. 1994.

He P, Zhu Q, Zhang Z, Zou X, Xu D. Relationship between the tibial mechanical axis and bony anatomical landmarks of the calf and foot measured on radiographs obtained with a new laser-calibrated position. *J Xray Sci Technol.* 2013;21(4):497–506. DOI: 10.3233/XST-130400.

Hirschmann A, Buck FM, Fucentese SF, Pfirrmann CW. Upright CT of the knee:the effect of weight-bearing on joint alignment. *Eur Radiol.* 2015;25 (11):3398–404. DOI: 10.1007/s00330-015-3756-6.

Hoad TF (ed). The concise Oxford dictionary of English etymology. Oxord, UK: *Oxford University Press.* 1996.

Hudek R, Schmutz S, Regenfelder F, Fuchs B, Koch PP. Novel measurement technique of the tibial slope on conventional MRI. *Clin Orthop Relat Res.* 2009;467:2066–72. DOI: 10.1007/s11999-009-0711-3.

Insall J, Salvati E. Patella position in the normal knee joint. *Radiology.* 1971;101(1):101–4. DOI: 10.1148/101.1.101.

Ioannidis JP. Why most discovered true associations are inflated. *Epidemiology.* 2008;19(5):640–8. DOI: 10.1097/EDE.0b013e31818131e7. *Erratum* in: *Epidemiology.* 2009; 20(4):629.

Irarrázaval S, Besa P, Fernández T, Fernández F, Donoso R, Tuca MJ, Lira MJ, Orrego M. Tibial tubercler to trochlear groove and the roman arch method for tibial tubercle lateralisation are reliable and distinguish between subjects with and without major patellar instability. *JISAKOS.* 2024; 9(3):272–8. DOI: 10.1016/j.jisako.2024.01.006.

Iseki T, Nakayama H, Daimon T, Kambara S, Kanto R, Yamaguchi M, Onishi S, Tachibana T, Yoshiya S. Tibial tubercle–midepicondyle distance can be a better index to predict the outcome of medial patellofemoral ligament reconstruction than tibial tubercle–trochlear groove distance. *Arthrosc Sports Med Rehab.* 2020;2(6):e697–704. DOI: 10.1016/j.asmr.2020.04.014.

Jones RB, Barlett EC, Vainright JR, Carroll RG. CT determination of tibial tubercle lateralization in patients presenting with anterior knee pain. *Skeletal Radiol.* 1995;24(7):505–9. DOI: 10.1007/BF00202146.

Judet J, Judet H, Massare C. Le scanner dans l'exploration des malpositions rotuliennes. [Use of the scanner for exploration of patella displacement (author's transl.)]. *Chirurgie*. 1979;105(7):535–9.

Keehan R, Gill A, Smith L, Ahmad R, Eldridge J. Mid inter-epicondyle trochlea intersection (MIELTI): proposal of a new index for identifying the deepest part of the trochlea. *Knee*. 2019;26(6):1204–9. DOI: 10.1016/j.knee.2019.10.011.

Kerby DS. The simple difference formula: an approach to teaching nonparametric correlation. *Innovative Teaching*. 2014;(3):1. DOI: 10.2466/11.IT.3.1.

Kirch W (ed). Encyclopedia of public health. Volume I. A–H. New York: *Springer*. 2008. DOI: 10.1007/978-1-4020-5614-7.

Knutsson F. Über die Röntgenologie des Femoropatellar-gelenks sowie eine gute Projektion für das Kniegelenk. 1941;371–6.

Krishnan H, Eldridge JD, Clark D, Metcalfe AJ, Stevens JM, Mandalia V. Tibial tuberosity–trochlear groove distance: does it measure up? *Bone Jt Open*. 2022;3–3:268–74. DOI:10.1302/2633-1462.33.BJO-2021-0107.

Li K, Xu C, Dong Z, Ji G, Wang F. Reliability of tibial tubercle–trochlear groove distance for assesing tibial tubercle lateralization: a study comparing different anatomic references. *Orthop J Sports Med*. 2024;12(4):23259671241239965. DOI: 10.1177/ 23259671241239965.

Lu Y, Fang JQ (eds). Advanced medical statistics. Singapore: *World Scientific Publishing Co*. 2003.

Matoničkin I, Erben R. Opća zoologija. Zagreb: *Školska knjiga*. 1994.

Miller PR, Klein RM, Teitge RA. Medial dislocation of the patella. *Skeletal Radiol*. 1991;20:429–31. DOI: 10.1007/BF00191085.

Moreland JR, Bassett LW, Hanker GJ. Radiographic analysis of the axial alignment of the lower extremity. *J Bone Joint Surg Am*. 1987;69-A(5):745–9.

Morris PE, Fritz CO. Why are effect sizes still neglected? *The Psychologist*. 2013;26:580–3.

Moya-Angeler J, Vairo GL, Bader DA, Sebastianelli WJ, Sherbondy PS. The tibial tubercle–trochlear groove distance/trochlear dysplasia index quotient is the most accurate indicator for determining patellofemoral instability risk. *Arthroscopy*. 2022;38(5):1608–14. DOI: 10.1016/j.arthro.2021.08.018.

Nizić D. Comparison of positions of the trochlear groove line and the vertical midline of the pericondylar rectangle on axial computed tomography: a retrospective pilot study. *Skeletal Radiol*. 2012;41(9):1099–104. DOI: 10.1007/s00256-011-1346-5.

Nizić D. The tibial tubercle–trochlear groove distance on axial CT and MRI: letter to the editor. *Am J Sports Med*. 2013; 41(12):NP53–4. DOI: 10.1177/0363546513512785.

Nizić D, Pervan M, Kovačević B. A new reference line in diagnosing a high-riding patella on routine digital lateral radiographs of the knee. *Skeletal Radiol*. 2014;43(8):1129–37. DOI: 10.1007/s00256-014-1825-6.

Nizić D, Šimunović M, Pavliša G, Jelić M. Tibial tuberosity–tibial intercondylar midpoint distance measured on computed tomography scanner is not biased during knee rotation and could be clinically more relevant than current measurement systems. *Int Orthop*. 2021;45(4):959–70. DOI: 10.1007/s00264-020-04820-6.

Nizić D, Šimunović M, Serdar J, Vlaić J, Josipović M, Levaj I, Ivić-Hofman I, Jelić M. Tibial tuberosity–tibial intercondylar midpoint distance can be interchangeably measured on axial CT and MRI: retrospective cross-sectional comparative study. *Medicina*. 2025;61(2):348–57. DOI: 10.3390/medicina61020348.

Nove-Josserand L, Dejour D. Dysplasie du qaudriceps et bascule rotulienne dans l'instabilité rotulienne objective [Quadriceps dysplasia and patellar tilt in objective patellar instability]. *Rev Chir Orthop Reparatrice Appar Mot.* 1995;81(6):497–504.

Paiva M, Blønd L, Hölmich P. Effect of medialization of the trochlear groove and lateralization of the tibial tubercle on TT-TG distance. A cross-sectional study of dysplastic and nondysplastic knees. *Am J Sports Med.* 2021;49(4):970–4. DOI: 10.1177/0363546520987819.

Paley D. Principles of deformity correction. 3rd ed. Heidelberg: *Springer.* 2002. DOI: 10.1007/978-3-642-59373-4.

Pascual-Leone N, Chipman D, Davie R, Bram BSJ, Mintz D, Fabricant P, Green D. Poster 285: MRI measurement of TT-TG can change without intervention: an analysis of sequential pre-operative MRIs in PFI patients. AOSSM Annual Meeting. *Orthop J Sports Med.* 2023;11(7; Suppl. 3). DOI: 10.1177/2325967123S00261.

Perez AR, Coladonato C, Sonnier JH, Saucedo ST, Avendano JP, Corvi J, Campbell M, Tjoumakaris FP, Cohen SB, Ciccotti MC, Freedman KB. Patients with first-time or recurrent patellar dislocations have a similar high rate and extent of articular cartilage injury observed on magnetic resonance imaging. *Arthrosc Sports Med Rehab.* 2024;6(1):100849. DOI: 10.1016/j.asmr.2023.100849.

Popper K. The logic of scientific discovery. London, New York: Routledge Classics (*Taylor & Francis Group*). 2005 (1959).

Rani S. Handbook of basic statistical concepts. For scientists and pharmacists. Oxord, UK: *Alpha Science International Ltd.* 2012.

Rosenthal R. Applied social research methods: meta-analytic procedures for social research. Thousand Oaks, CA: *SAGE Publications Ltd.* 1991. DOI: 10.4135/9781412984997.

Schäfer T, Schwarz MA. The meaningfulness of effect sizes in psychological research: differences between subdisciplines and the impact of potential biases. *Front Psychol.* 2019;10:813. DOI: 10.3389/fpsyg.2019.00813.

Schmidt FL. Statistical significance testing and cumulative knowledge in psychology: implications for training of researches. *Psychological methods*. 1996;1:115–29.

Seitlinger G, Scheurecker G, Högler R, Labey L, Innocenti B, Hofmann S. Tibial tubercle–posterior cruciate ligament distance: a new measurement to define the position of the tibial tubercle in patients with patellar dislocation. *Am J Sports Med.* 2012;40(5):1119–25. DOI: 10.1177/0363546512438762.

Serdar V. Udžbenik statistike. Zagreb: *Školska knjiga*. 1966.

Shrout PE, Fleiss JL. Intraclass correlations: uses in assessing rater reliability. *Psychol Bull*. 1979;86(2):420–8. DOI: 10.1037//0033-2909.86.2.420.

Stangroom J. Social science statistics. Available at: *https://www.socscistatistics.com*. 24.2.2025.;17:05.

Šimunović M. Povezanost površine poprečnoga presjeka *musculus vastus medialis obliquus* i vrijednosti postraničnoga nagiba patele kod instabiliteta patelofemoralnoga zgloba. Disertacija. [Correlation of the cross-sectional area of the *vastus medialis obliquus* muscle and the value of the lateral patellar tilt in patellofemoral instability]. Zagreb: *Sveučilište u Zagrebu, Medicinski fakultet*. 2023. Available at: *https://urn.nsk.hr/urn:nbn:hr:105:869122*.

Šošić I. Primijenjena statistika. Zagreb: *Školska knjiga*. 2004.

Tan SHS, Lim BY, Chng KSJ, Doshi C, Wong FKL, Lim AKS, Hui JH. The difference between computed tomography and magnetic resonance imaging mesurements of tibial tubercle–trochlear groove distance for patients with or without patellofemoral instability: a systematic review and meta-analysis. *J Knee Surg*. 2020;33(8):768–76. DOI: 10.1055/s-0039-1688563.

Targ S. Theoretical mechanics. A short course. Moscow: *Mir Publishers*. 1988.

Tavernier T, Dejour D. Imagerie du genou: quel examen choisir? *Encycl Méd Chir*. (Editions Scientifiques et Médicales Elsevier SAS, Paris, tous droits réservés), Radiodiagnostic – Squelette normal. 2001;30-433-A-20:1–18.

Tscholl PM, Antoniadis A, Dietrich TJ, Koch PP, Fucentese SF. The tibial tubercle–trochlear groove distance in patients with trochlear dysplasia: the influence of the proximally flat trochlea. *Knee Surg Sports Traumatol Arthrosc.* 2016;24(9):2741–7. DOI: 10.1007/S00167-014-3386-6.

Wilcoxon F. Individual comparisons by ranking methods. *Biometrics Bulletin.* 1945;1(6):80–3. DOI: 10.2307/3001968.

Xu Z, Zhang H, Fu B, Mohamed SI, Zhang J, Zhou A. Tibial tubercle–Roman arch distance: a new measurement of patellar dislocation and indication of tibial tubercle osteotomy. *Orthop J Sports Med.* 2020;8(4):2325967120914872. DOI: 10.1177/2325967120914872.

7

Index

terms & people

Numbers in *italic* indicate a page with a figure.

Index

A — a

E — e

F — f

G — g

H — h

I — i

K — k

L — l

M — m

Index

R — r

T — t

V — v

Index

Z — z

8

Glossary

of important terms

Glossary

95 % confidence interval: the interval calculated from the measured values having 95 % probability that the unknown parameter lies *within* the interval

accuracy: the closeness of the measured value and the true value

bias: the error with regard to the ways the targeted and sampled populations are different; it undermines the validity of a study

closure (rectification): according to the *Gestalt* theory of human perception, an ability to perceive *incomplete* forms as *complete* using an *a priori* familiar shape such as the triangle, rectangle, and alike

confounder: a variable affecting either the indicator or the condition thereby changing the outcome; a 'nuisance' variable

critical value: the value a test must *exceed* in order for the null-hypothesis to be rejected

cut: a transverse (axial) CT image | **'headless'** ~ when scrolling in the caudo-cranial direction, the first transverse (axial) CT image where the top of the fibular head was no longer visible • **'prominent'**

~ when scrolling in the cranio-caudal direction, the transverse (axial) CT image where the tibial tuberosity was the most prominent, that is to say the most *anterior* • **reference** ~ a cut used for measurement at different knees/legs • **'6-~'** a cut used for measurement of the transverse diameter of the quadriceps belly as the 30th cranial CT image from the CT image on which the patella was no longer visible (30 × 2 mm = 60 mm = 6 cm)

cut-off: a border value between negatives and positives | **true** ~ the population mean of a variable

distance: a line between two points; in this small CT study, a line in the frontal plane between the medial point, reflecting the relative middle of the knee/leg (trochlear groove point or the tibial intercondylar midpoint) and the lateral point, reflecting the quadricep muscle insertion (the tibial tuberosity point); measured in the transverse (axial) plane

dysplasia: an irregular formation; in this small CT study, used with regard to the *femoral trochlea* (*femoral trochlear* ~) to indicate an irregular bone relief of the femoral trochlear groove with a simple four-type gradation system by Tavernier and Dejour from mild (types A and B) to severe (types C and D) forms

error: | **type I** ~ rejecting a true null-hypothesis or detecting a non-existent difference • **type II** ~ not rejecting a false null-hypothesis or not detecting an existant difference • **type M ~ (exaggeration ratio)** a phenomenon where the magnitude for a relationship of interest is *large* and statistically significant in *smaller* samples, yet becomes *small* and statistically significant in *larger* samples (the magnitude *deflates*)

indicator: a variable indicating a condition

integer: a whole number

magnitude: the size of an effect

mean: the sum of values divided by the total of values (in the population or in the sample)

mechanism: a collection of material points (particles) or bodies in which the position or motion of *each* particle or body of the system depends on the position and motion of *all* the other particles or bodies | **quadriceps (muscle) ~** a four-part mechanism for leg extension in the knee joint, consisting of the *origin*, the *belly* ('quadriceps' meaning 'four heads' in Latin), the superior and inferior part of the *tendon* enclosing the *patella*, and the *insertion* (the tibial tuberosity)

median: the middle value (in the population or in the sample), dividing the distribution in half

modality: type of imaging (ultrasound, X-rays, CT and MRI)

orthogonal coordinate (Cartesian) system: an imaginary composition of three mutually perpendicular planes (frontal, transverse, and sagittal) in which a position of a *movable* point is referred to with regard to the *immovable* center (the origin); used extensively in radiologic imaging

outcome: the result of a study

P value: the probability of detecting a result *equally or more* extreme than the one detected by chance

precision: consistency of repeated results

prevalence: a proportion of *positives* in the sample

receiver operating characteristic (curve): a ratio between a false positive rate and a true positive rate for a given test; compares two tests for accuracy *without* knowing their cut-offs

reliability: consistency of a measurement instrument | **test-retest** ~ a measure of the degree to which an instrument provides a consistent measure of a characteristic on different occasions

resolution: the *smallest* change of the measurement value that a measurement instrument can show

rotation: a circular motion *around* an axis

sensitivity: a proportion of correctly detected *positives*

Spearman's rank correlation coefficient (rho): a nonparametric correlation coefficient measuring the tendency of two measurements to vary together

specificity: a proportion of correctly detected *negatives*

standard deviation: the square root of the average of the squared deviations of the observations from their mean; it tells you how far away is the measured value from the mean on average; the lower the standard deviation, the higher the precision

strain: a longitudinal dilatation of a prismatic bar under axial weight-bearing conditions (*tendon* ~)

symmetric distribution (and curve): a distribution with *equal* shape on both sides of the mean where mean, median and mode are *equal*; it is often called *normal*, *bell-shaped* or *Gaussian*

test: a method of distinguishing the negatives and the positives with accuracy (sensitivity and specificity) *above* 50 %, as opposed to *guessing* | **diagnostic** ~ an imaging test with *low* sensitivity and *high* specificity, excels in detecting *negatives* • **screening** ~ an imaging test with *high* sensitivity and *low* specificity, excels in detecting *positives* • **statistical** ~ a calculus used to test a null-hypothesis • **Wilcoxon signed-rank** ~ a nonparametric statistical test comparing two *dependent* samples with *ordinal* or *numerical* measured values having *nonsymmetric* distribution (or where symmetric distribution cannot be guaranteed)

translation: a linear motion *along* an axis

validity: the ability to measure the characteristic of interest | **sorting** ~ the ability to distinguish the positives and negatives • **tracking** ~ the ability to track the therapy success

variable: a qualitative or quantitative characteristic of interest exhibiting different values in different study units; a changeable value of interest

variance: the square of standard deviation
yaw: a rotation around *z*-axis

9

The Author

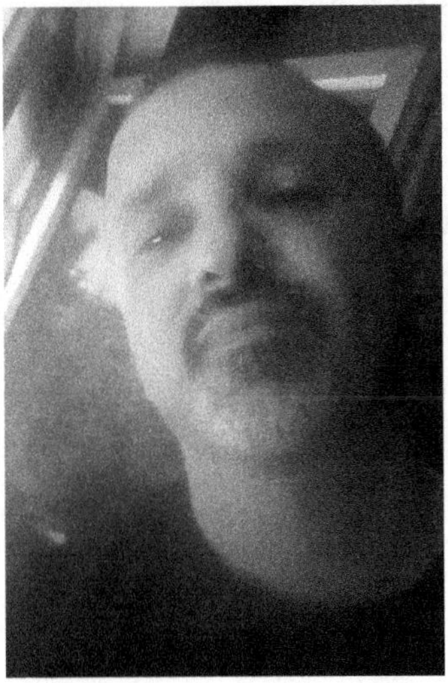

Dinko Nizić (born 16th December 1978, Slavonski Brod, Republic of Croatia) is a radiologist and a published scientific author in the field of patellofemoral instability. He graduated at the *Medical Faculty of Osijek* at the *Josip Juraj Strossmayer University* in 2005, and finished his residency as well as radiology training in 2014 at the *University Hospital Center Zagreb*. From 2015 to 2023 he was the head of the *Department of Radiology and Ultrasound Diagnostics* in the *Special hospital for pulmonary diseases* in Zagreb, working as a freelance radiologist since.

He received his PhD at the University of Zagreb in 2024. Until now, he has published many scientific publications indexed in the international databases. According to the full list of publications in the *Google Scholar* database (https://scholar.google.com/citations?hl=en&user=Llse7kgAAAAJ&view_op=list_works) on 2025-09-29 he has been cited over 220 times (*h*-index = 8, *i10*-index = 8).

He is a member of various Croatian and foreign expert societies.

Notes

Notes